Nurses' Aids Series

PRACTICAL PROCEDURES FOR NURSES

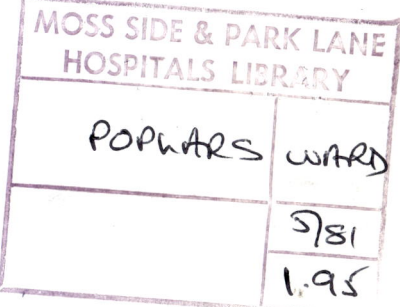
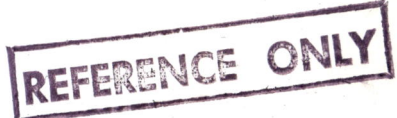

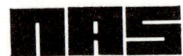

NURSES' AIDS SERIES

Nurses' Aids Series

Practical Procedures for Nurses

Second Edition

DORIS H. M. BILLING
S.R.N., R.C.N.T.,
Pupil Nurse Teacher at the Peterborough District Hospital

BAILLIÈRE TINDALL LONDON

A BAILLIÈRE TINDALL book published by
Cassell Ltd.
35 Red Lion Square, London WC1R 4SG
and at Sydney, Auckland, Toronto, Johannesburg
an affiliate of
Macmillan Publishing Company Inc.
New York

First published as *Tray and Trolley Setting* by Marjorie Houghton, 1941
    Sixth edition, 1960. Reprinted four times
Published as *Practical Procedures for Nurses* by Marjorie Houghton and
    J. E. Parnell, 1969
    Reprinted 1972
Published as *Practical Procedures for Nurses*, Second edition, by
    Doris H. M. Billing, 1976
Reprinted 1979

ISBN 0 7020 0604 1

© 1976 Baillière Tindall

Set, printed and bound in Great Britain by
Cox & Wyman Ltd
London, Fakenham and Reading

Contents

Preface

Over the years, many new practical nursing textbooks have been published, but, in a library used by nurses, there is always a place for a book which provides a guide for recognition of instruments, and preparation for the carrying out of procedures.

Nursing is essentially a practical subject and therefore the nurse needs to be able to apply the knowledge and skills she has acquired to the ward situation.

In 1940, Miss M. Houghton prepared the book known as *Aids to Tray and Trolley Setting*, her objective being to present various procedures in such a way as to enable the nurse to understand clearly and simply the settings required for ward and out-patient department procedures. That she was successful became evident by the popularity of the book, so much so, that in 1967, Miss Houghton, together with Miss J. E. Parnell, reconstructed the book to keep abreast of current patterns in nurse education. When published in 1968 the book was entitled *Practical Procedures for Nurses* and once again, its popularity became widespread.

Bearing in mind the success of the book in the past, it was not without trepidation that I approached the task of its revision.

This latest edition is designed to meet modern trends in nursing and to encourage the nurse to remember, in an orderly manner, the necessary equipment for the setting of a tray or trolley, whilst remembering that hospitals throughout the country and, indeed, throughout the world have widely varying needs in a book on this subject.

My thanks are extended to my colleagues in all wards and

departments of the District Hospital, Peterborough and in particular to my fellow members of the staff of the College of Education. Special thanks are due to Miss J. Burbage, for her unfailing advice and help throughout the preparation of the texts, and Mr J. Pitts for the considerable time and patience he devoted to the photographs included in the book. I must also add my thanks to the publishers, who helped and encouraged me.

I gratefully acknowledge permission to reproduce photographs and illustrations provided by the following producers of medical equipment: Downs Surgical Ltd, Gillette Surgical, Pharmax Ltd, Portex Ltd, Sandoz Products Ltd, Scholl Ltd, Sherwood Medical Industries Ltd, Simpla Plastics Ltd, Smith & Nephew Pharmaceuticals Ltd, Travenol Laboratories Ltd, Vickers Medical Ltd, Warne Surgical Products Ltd.

January 1976   D. H. M. BILLING

1 Preparation of the Patient

The preparation of a patient for any procedure, no matter how trivial, should be considered carefully by the nurse before contemplating any form of action, and can best be considered under two main headings: Psychological and Physical.

Psychological

This may, in fact, be the patient's first experience of hospital. First impressions begin either as soon as a notice is received of pending admission, if it is a routine planned admission, or as soon as the doors of the accident and emergency department are entered, if an emergency admission.

Patients frequently enter hospitals, having no idea of the routine or who's who, and it is therefore of great importance that all grades of hospital staff realize the need to greet patients and distraught relatives with kindness and courtesy at all times.

The nurse should always remember that no matter how trivial an illness or operation may seem to her, it is a milestone in the life of the patient, and to the family, a major upheaval. A mother may be leaving behind small children in the care of relatives or friends, or a man may be receiving considerably reduced financial benefits and an elderly person may have had to leave an aged partner. These matters constitute a worry to the patient. Today's hospitals provide help to dispel such worries and so leave the patient with a more contented mind which can benefit the physical condition.

It is of the utmost importance that the nurse quickly

discovers the patient's name and addresses him by it. To be a bed number or described by one's condition is humiliating.

When Florence Nightingale commenced her nursing school, she stressed to her nurses that 'the hospital should do the patient no harm'; this, I am sure applies mentally as well as physically.

Physical

There is no greater fear than that of the unknown, so the nurse should always, before commencing any procedure, tell the patient exactly what she is going to do and how he can best cooperate. To gain the patient's cooperation and confidence is halfway to accomplishing even the most difficult and unpleasant task.

The next consideration when performing any physical preparation, should be the patient's comfort and privacy. A patient cannot cooperate with the nurse fully if he wishes to use a bed pan, urinal or if he is sitting uncomfortably in bed. Neither can he cooperate if he is suffering embarrassment through being exposed. The nurse should never find it necessary to expose more of the patient than the area she is treating or the area that is being examined. The screens round the patient's bed should be drawn with care as the treatment is something personal to the patient and the nurse and not an experience to be shared with the remainder of the people in the ward.

A good guide for nurses is to try to put themselves in the position of the patient or the relatives and think, 'Would I like this to happen to me?'

2   Preparation of Equipment

This book deals with the preparation for various procedures, investigations and examinations commonly carried out in the wards or the out-patient departments of the hospital, and for which the nurse is responsible. The illustrations provide a guide to the equipment needed and the text indicates the reasons for a particular procedure and any special points in the preparation and care of the patient. It may be thought that such a presentation overemphasizes the technical side of the nurse's work, but technical efficiency is a part of good nursing care. Valuable time can be saved and the patient's comfort promoted if the nurse knows what is wanted and the preparation required in each case. Indeed, the patient's safety, and in an emergency his life, may depend on the nurse's ability to anticipate and to provide, ready for immediate use, all the items required for any likely procedure.

There are, of course, methods and types of apparatus in use other than those depicted in this book, but in each case the procedure described can be efficiently carried out with the equipment illustrated.

With the advent of new materials, particularly plastics, new methods of packaging and sterilization have been introduced in many hospitals with consequent changes in the details of some techniques. However, the basic principles in the conduct of surgical dressings and other sterile procedures remain:

1. The prevention of contamination wherever possible.
2. The conscientious and meticulous performance of the process of cleaning and sterilization, whether manual or automatic.

3. Proper handling of sterile material.
4. Distinction between sterile and merely clean articles.

In circumstances where cost is not considered an important factor, almost all equipment, from bed pans and other utensils to surgeon's gloves and complete packs for all sterile procedures, is disposable. In other hospitals disposable face masks, dressing towels, single use intravenous sets, syringes, needles and catheters are in general use, but other articles such as instruments, bowls and gallipots are cleaned and resterilized. In many developing countries where modernization and expansion of the hospital service is often limited by the money available, capital outlay for a complete Central Sterile Supply Service and disposable equipment cannot be found. In such circumstances central packing and sterilization of as much equipment as possible should be aimed at in order that sterilization processes can be controlled and economy in the use of some items effected.

Sterilization

Sterilization in the surgical sense means that all living micro-organisms have been destroyed. Sterility is required when any incision or puncture of the skin is to be made, when wounds require dressing or when any instrument is to be introduced into a body cavity or passage which is normally sterile, e.g. the urinary bladder. Domestic cleanliness, but not surgical sterility, is adequate for apparatus such as that used for enemas, where there is little danger of introducing infection. All such non-sterile equipment, unless disposable, must be thoroughly cleaned and boiled after use.

Before any article is subjected to the process of sterilization it must first be cleaned. Organic material, such as blood or serum for example, left on instruments will form a barrier to effective sterilization, unless a modern, high speed, high vacuum autoclave, with its ability to transmit heat by conduction, is used. In Central Sterile Supply Departments cleaning of instruments is usually carried out by automatic washing machines. In the wards scrubbing with soap and water is the usual method with special attention being paid to hinges and serrated blades of forceps. Glass syringes and non-disposable needles which have been used for the withdrawal of blood or serum are more easily cleaned if put into cold disinfectant solution after use. Rubber tubing, rubber and gum elastic catheters are difficult to clean; cold water should be run through them from both ends followed by washing in hot soapy water and rinsing. When cleaning very fine tubing or catheters, water should be forced through from both ends, with a syringe. Gum elastic has a further disadvantage in being easily damaged by heat and also needs very careful handling. Sterilization is normally carried out by exposing the material to the vapour given off by paraformaldehyde tablets in a closed container. Under no circumstances should this container be placed on a hot surface, as the resultant fumes are highly toxic. Plastic tubing and catheters which are only used once are increasingly replacing these materials. Plastic funnels and connectors are useful for many purposes in place of glass, which is so easily broken.

When dealing with delicate instruments such as the various types of endoscope, the nurse should find out the method of cleaning and sterilizing to be followed in each case. Sigmoidoscopes and cystoscopes, for example are taken apart for cleaning, carefully washed in warm soapy water and rinsed. Some parts of these instruments such as metal sheaths and obturators can be boiled for five minutes and then dried. Optical parts and lights may be damaged by boiling due to the destruction of the holding cement. Any aqueous disinfectant fluid (except phenol compounds) may be used. Long immersion should be avoided. However some cytoscopes are completely boilable, even autoclaveable, and in every case the nurse should obtain exact instructions and follow them carefully.

Methods of Sterilization

In hospital practice heat is the usual sterilizing agent. Heat is most effective in the form of steam under pressure or hot air at high temperature. Boiling is not an effective means of sterilization. Vegetative organisms are readily killed by exposure to boiling water, but spore-forming organisms are only killed at considerably higher temperatures which can only be achieved either by the modern autoclave or dry heat method.

Autoclaving   Sterilization by steam under pressure and at high temperature is the process known as autoclaving. The autoclave consists of a stout steel jacket with a door or lid which can be firmly fixed by clamps and an inner chamber in which the articles to be sterilized are placed. The older type of autoclave is hand-operated. The new high-speed high-vacuum autoclaves are entirely automatic and air is removed by a vacuum pump. When the autoclave has been loaded and the door closed, air is first extracted from the apparatus and steam is then admitted. The steam must be dry and under pressure if sterilization is to be attained. Under these conditions steam will condense when it meets the cooler temperature of the articles in the autoclave and the latent heat released will penetrate and kill any living organisms. The minimum time required for the destruction of all living organisms depends on the temperature and pressure reached in the autoclave chamber, as will be seen from the following examples:

Temperature	Pressure (bars)	Minimum sterilizing time
134 °C (273 °F)	2·00	3 min
126 °C (259 °F)	1·35	10 min
121 °C (250 °F)	1·00	15 min

The automatic high-speed autoclave is preset and cannot be adjusted. Articles to be autoclaved are packaged in paper or cotton cloth wrappings or, less and less frequently, packed in metal drums. In the latter case it is necessary to make sure that the drum lids are fitting properly, that the shutters covering the holes in the sides are open when the drums are put into the autoclave (otherwise steam cannot meet the materials inside) and that they are closed before the drums are removed from the autoclave. Bulk packaging of dressings in drums is not a safe practice as it may result in the drum being opened several times during the course of the day to remove part of its contents, giving rise to inevitable contamination. Single dressing packs are safer. Whatever method is used, articles must not be packed tightly in their containers and the autoclave must not be overloaded, for in either case the steam will not be able to penetrate through the articles to be sterilized, especially in older manual machines.

Autoclaving is suitable for the sterilization of textile materials, paper (such as paper towels, masks, caps and gowns), most instruments, metal, rubber and glass articles and some types of plastic materials. Tests for the efficiency of sterilization are carried out at regular intervals, usually under the direction of the bacteriologist. These tests include the use of colour indicators and bacteriological tests.

Dry heat Sterilization by dry heat is effective if the articles are exposed to a sufficiently high temperature for a sufficient time. A temperature of not less than 160 °C (320 °F) is required in the hot air oven and the articles should be exposed to this temperature for one hour. This is a useful method for equipment which deteriorates in steam, e.g. laboratory glassware and all-glass syringes. Hot air is also used for sterilizing some instruments, e.g. ophthalmic instruments, to prevent water erosion of cutting edges.

Boiling   Boiling water tank sterilizers are still in general use in many hospitals for the sterilization of instruments and bowls and, under proper conditions, boiling is a 'reasonably' safe method. If the water is made alkaline by the addition of sodium carbonate, forming a 2 % solution, the lethal effect on bacteria is increased. If rubber articles such as tubing, catheters or gloves are boiled, no soda should be added to the water. The conditions which are necessary for efficient sterilization by boiling are:

1. The sterilizer must be properly packed; if articles such as bowls lie one inside each other, or upside down, pockets of air will be formed and the heat cannot penetrate effectively.

2. All articles must be completely immersed in the water.

3. The water should be boiling when the instruments are put in (except where the article to be sterilized would be damaged by immersion in boiling water and must therefore be put into cooler water which is then brought to the boil).

4. The water must boil again after the articles are put in before timing the period of sterilization.

Although two minutes boiling will kill all organisms in the vegetative form, it is the usual practice to boil for five minutes, thus allowing a good margin of safety. If contamination with resistant spore-bearers is suspected, then either autoclaving or repeated, prolonged boiling, rapid cooling, boiling, is necessary. The articles are boiled for one hour then cooled rapidly by immersing in cold water and boiled again for a further hour. Any spores that were not killed in the first boiling are likely to revert to the vegetative form during the cooling process and these will then be killed during the second boiling.

Gamma radiation from a radioactive source is used commercially for the sterilization of many prepacked sterile articles such as plastic catheters, intravenous sets, suture materials, knife blades. This type of sterilization is very useful for equipment which cannot be effectively treated by heat without damage, but it is not a method which can be used in the hospital. Use may be made of this method through the 'packet' system of the United Kingdom Atomic Energy Authority.

Chemical disinfection is used mainly as an adjunct to other methods of sterilization. For example, where bowl and instrument handling forceps are used, these instruments are first sterilized by boiling and then kept in tall jars containing a disinfectant solution such as Stericol 1:100 solution.

Disinfectants are also used in the treatment of infected textile materials such as bed linen, gowns, masks and infants' napkins, although the modern hospital laundry is equipped to deal with infected linen and soaking in disinfectant is therefore unnecessary. As skin cleaning agents the cationic detergents such as Hibitane and Savlon, which remove grease from the skin and with it the dirt and bacteria on the surface, are useful. It should be noted that skin is never regarded as 'sterile'. Although the hands must be washed and 'socially clean' before any sterile procedure is undertaken, handling of sterile material is done entirely with sterilized forceps unless the operator's hands are covered by sterile gloves.

The following table gives a list of some of the commoner disinfectants and antiseptics and their use:

Substance	Uses	Strength
Benzalkonium chloride (Roccal)	Disinfection of skin	1:10 solution
	Disinfection of linen and utensils, also deodorant	1:40 solution
Chloroxylenol and similar preparations, e.g. Dettol and Osyl	These preparations are less irritating and less caustic than phenol or cresol	
	Disinfection of linen and utensils	1:20 to 1:40 solution
	Antiseptic hand lotion	1:40 to 1:100 solution
Chlorhexidine (Hibitane)	Skin disinfection. Disinfection of instruments and working surfaces	0·5% in 70% spirit
Chlorine in the form of hypochlorite solutions, e.g. eusol, electrolytic hypochlorit (Milton)	As a dressing or irrigating lotion in the treatment of sloughing or infected tissues	
	For disinfection and storage of infants' feeding bottles and utensils	1:80 solution
Flavine group: acriflavine, proflavine, euflavine and 5-aminoacridine	These dyes are used in the treatment of wounds and as antiseptics on the skin. They may be combined with sterile liquid paraffin as an oily dressing	1:1000 solution in water or spirit (proflavine is not soluble in spirit)
Formaldehyde and formalin (a solution of formaldehyde in water)	For disinfecting articles which cannot be treated with steam, e.g. books and leather articles; for fumigation of rooms	If used as a spray, 240 ml formalin to 4l water for every 36m^2 of surface
Paraform tablets which disintegrate slowly, liberating formaldehyde	For the sterilization and storage of elastic gum articles and endoscopes	
Hydrogen peroxide	Used for the irrigation of wounds and cleaning septic mouth conditions. Is non-poisonous and in the presence of organic matter readily liberates oxygen and helps in the separation of sloughs	Stock solutions contain 10 or 20 vol. of available oxygen. Diluted with warm water, as required, in 2·5, 5 or 10 volumes
Iodine	Used for skin preparation, it is more penetrating than most skin paints especially if the skin is dry	'Weak tincture of iodine' 1:40
Iodine solution (Povidone)	Used for skin preparation and in the treatment of wounds	1% of available iodine
Mercurial preparations: phenylmercuric nitrate	Used for sterilizing certain instruments, e.g. the telescopes and sheaths of non-boilable cystoscopes; for preserving fluids and suspensions prepared for parenteral injection	1:2000 to 1:10000 solution
	For skin preparation	
	As a vaginal douche for non-specific infections	
	For mycotic infections	$\frac{1}{2}$ or 1:1000 in a water soluble ointment base

Substance	Uses	Strength
Phenol (carbolic acid)	Liquefied phenol, carbolic acid *poisonous and corrosive*, if splashed on the skin should be swabbed off at once with methylated or surgical spirit	
	Disinfecting linen, crockery and sanitary utensils	1:20
	Disinfecting excreta	1:10 for 1 h
Crude phenolic disinfectants, i.e. 'black' and 'white' disinfecting fluids, e.g. Jeyes fluid, Cyllin, Izal	Disinfecting excreta	1:10 solution mixed with excreta for 2 h
	Disinfecting linen ('white' fluids should be used as 'black' fluids may stain linen)	1:160 solution for 12 h
	Scrubbing floors, laboratory or sluice room benches, etc.	1:160 solution
	For local pollution of floors, e.g. with sputum	Swab with 1:5 solution
Savlon (0·3% chlorhexidine with 3% cetrimide)	Skin cleansing	1:20 solution
Sodium chloride solutions:		
Normal saline (Physiological Solution of Sodium Chloride B.P.)	Used for bathing and irrigating wounds and cavities: for rectal, subcutaneous, and intravenous injection	9:1000 solution
Hypertonic salt solution	In the treatment of wounds as baths or irrigations	1 to 2:10 solution
Glutaraldehyde solution	Used for sterilizing certain instruments, e.g. endoscopes	1:50 solution
	For rubber or plastic equipment	

3　Sterile Procedures

Preparation of the Dressing Trolley

Before and after the procedure, the trolley is thoroughly washed with soap and water and dried. If desired, the trolley may also be mopped with a suitable antiseptic, such as 0·5 % chlorhexidine in 70 % spirit. The general rule in setting a trolley for a sterile procedure is that the sterile articles are placed on the top shelf and unsterile articles on the bottom.

In some hospitals it is customary to cover the trolley with a sterile sheet of impermeable material. The sterile equipment is then placed directly on this and covered with a sterile towel.

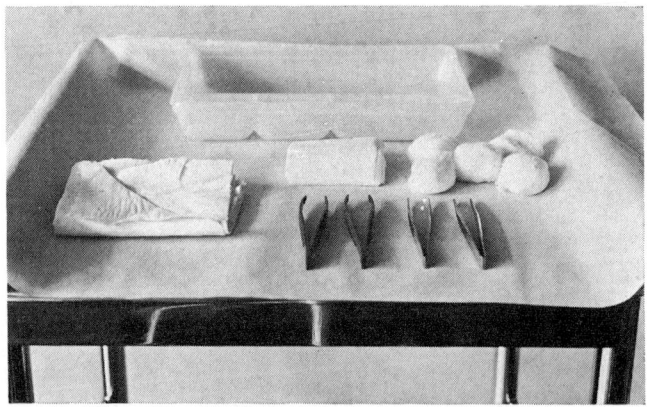

FIG. 1. Basic dressing pack opened out

Preparation of the Hands of the Operator

Hands can never be regarded as sterile and therefore all sterilized instruments and materials which will come into contact with the wound or with any puncture of the skin surface are handled with sterile forceps. The only exception to this is when the hands are covered by sterilized gloves. However, the hands of the dresser and the assistant should be washed before beginning the procedure and, since wet hands are more likely to convey bacteria than dry ones, dried on a clean towel. Damp towels which have been used several times are a possible source of infection and, for this reason, many hospitals use disposable paper towels. If these are not available there should be an adequate supply of clean dry towels.

The Use of Face Masks

In many hospitals the wearing of face masks while carrying out surgical dressings is no longer routine practice. If masks are used they should be worn only while actually carrying out the procedure and then discarded. Disposable paper masks are suitable for use for short periods.

Surgical Dressings

Basic Equipment for Surgical Dressings and Other Sterile Procedures

Where a Central Sterile Supply Service provides all the necessary equipment in sterile packs, the following items will be needed:

Top shelf of the dressing trolley (when in use)

Sterile pack or packs containing:

Paper dressing towel

Wool mops and dressing materials, e.g. folded gauze, cotton wool

1 gallipot

4 pairs plain dissecting forceps or dressing forceps

1 pair of scissors (which may be included with the other instruments or supplied in a separate pack).

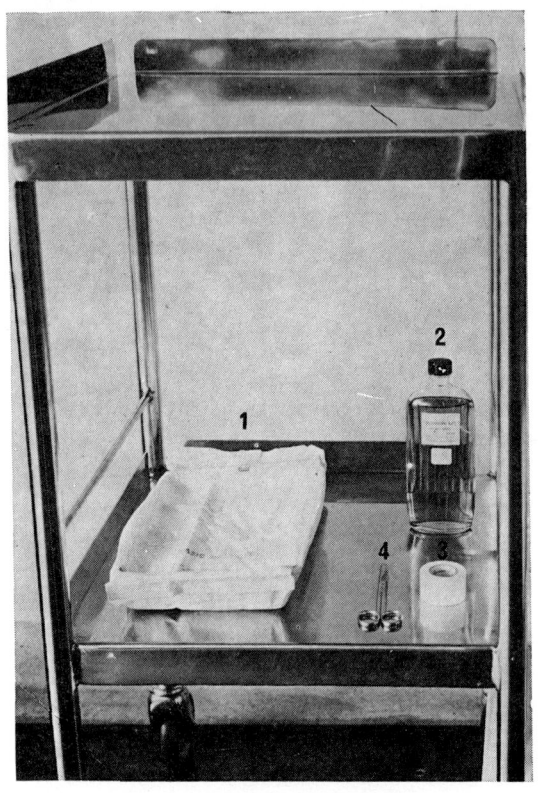

FIG. 2. A dressing trolley

1. Basic dressing pack containing: paper dressing towel; forceps; gauze; cotton wool; and gallipots

2. Lotion

3. Strapping

4. Scissors

Bottom shelf of the dressing trolley

Bandages, safety pins, scissors, adhesive tape, Nobecutane

Lotion for skin cleaning, e.g. 0·5 % chlorhexidine in 70 % spirit

Methylated ether or other solvents may be needed to remove strapping marks, or Nobecutane.

Extra packs which might be needed are usually placed on the bottom shelf of the trolley.

Disposal of soiled equipment Soiled dressings may be placed in a paper bag attached to the lower rail of the trolley and later transferred to a bin. If no bags are available, the dressings are discarded into a foot-operated pedal bin.

Used instruments may also be discarded into a paper bag attached to the lower rail of the trolley.

If there is no Central Sterile Supply Service in operation, all sterile equipment is prepared in the ward and the following items are needed:

Top shelf

Sterile bowl containing the sterile pack of dressings and a towel

Sterile gallipot

Sterile instrument dish containing four pairs of plain dissecting forceps or dressing forceps and scissors.

Bottom shelf

The items needed, are listed for the trolley setting as given above.

Additional items to be added to the top shelf of the trolley for removal of stitches or clips

1 pair sterile sharp-pointed stitch scissors or disposable stitch cutter

1 pair sterile Michel's clip-removing forceps.

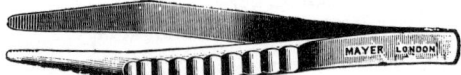

FIG. 3. Plain dissecting forceps

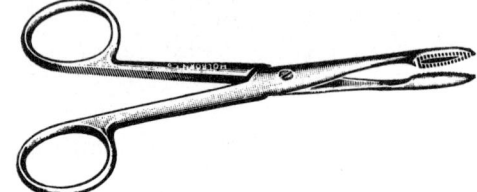

FIG. 4. French pattern dressing forceps

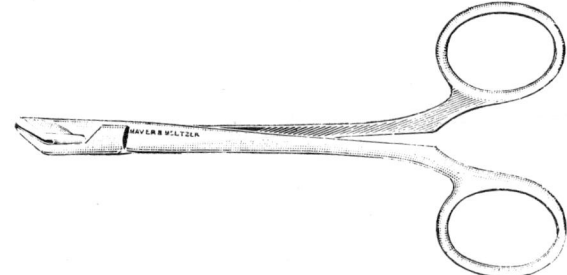

FIG. 5. Michel's clip-removing forceps

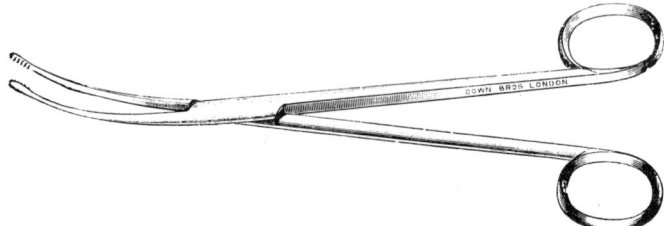

FIG. 6. Lister's curved sinus forceps

FIG. 7. Wound probe

Additional items to be added to the top shelf of the trolley for exploration of a wound

1 pair sterile sinus forceps
1 sterile probe
Sterile ribbon gauze—usually 6 mm width
1 sterile gallipot for solution if ordered for use with ribbon gauze.

Equipment for Special Investigations and Treatments in the Ward

The following sterile basic equipment should be added to that listed for surgical dressings:

Top shelf
2 dressing towels
2 gallipots
Packs or sterile instrument dish containing:
1 pair blunt-ended scissors
1 Bard-Parker knife handle
Selection of Bard-Parker blades
Syringes and needles for local anaesthetic, e.g. 2 ml and 5 ml syringes and needles sizes 17 and 20.

Bottom shelf
Bottles of an iodine preparation for skin marking, and collodion
Local anaesthetic, e.g. lignocaine 1 or 2 % solution
Sterile containers for specimens of fluid or tissue
Pathology request forms and labels.

Injection tray with stimulants A selection of sterile 1 ml syringes and needles for hypodermic or intramuscular injection of drugs should be to hand. In some hospitals it is the practice to include a stimulant tray on the bottom shelf of the trolley. Ampoules of drugs likely to be needed and the patient's prescription sheet should be immediately available.

If the area of the patient's bed is not well lit then an Angle-poise lamp should be provided. A small blanket or shawl may be necessary to keep the patient warm during the procedure.

Equipment to shave the skin should be available for use; obvious hairs must be removed from an area of intact skin through which sterile equipment is to be introduced into the body.

Tracheostomy

Tracheostomy is the operation of making an opening into the trachea and inserting a tube through which the patient can breathe. This procedure is normally carried out in the operating theatre. If, in an emergency, it is to be performed in the ward, a sterile pack can often be obtained from the theatre and will usually contain the equipment as given in the list below.

In an acute and unforeseen emergency, a tray containing a sterile Bard-Parker handle carrying a pointed blade, a pair of sterile tracheal dilators or, as a substitute, a pair of dressing forceps, will enable the operator to make an opening through which the patient can breathe while the tracheostomy tube and other equipment is being obtained.

In addition to the equipment for special investigation as listed on pages 17–18 (specimen containers not required), sterile packs or instrument dishes should be added, containing the following sterile equipment:

Top shelf
  6 towel clips
  2 dressing towels
  Additional gauze mops
  1 pair toothed dissecting forceps
  1 pair non-toothed dissecting forceps
  2 pairs sponge holding forceps
  4 pairs fine tissue forceps, e.g. Allis's
  1 pair each of long and short curved scissors
  8 pairs artery forceps (2 Spencer Wells', 6 fine 'mosquito'—
Kelly's)
  1 blunt hook
  1 sharp hook
  2 double hook retractors
  Tracheal dilators
  Tracheostomy tubes and introducers
  Tape
  Black thread, e.g. 2/0

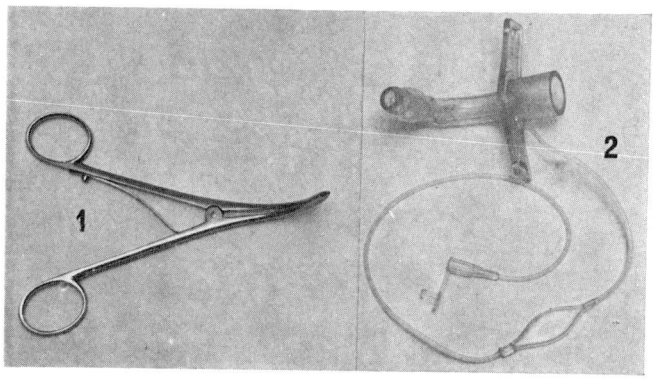

FIG. 8.

1. Tracheal dilator
2. Bassett's cuffed Portex tracheostomy tube

Half-circle cutting edge suture needles, e.g. 2 each of sizes 12 and 14

Needle holder

Suction apparatus and 2 suction catheters.

Bottom shelf

Add a sandbag to be placed high under the shoulders to extend the patient's neck.

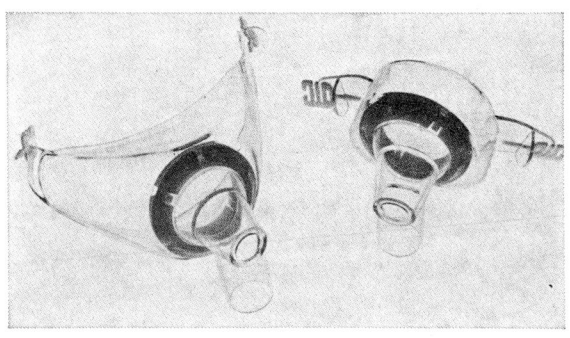

Fig. 9. Adult and paediatric tracheostomy masks
for the administration of oxygen

Care of the Patient

After a tracheostomy, the following should be ready for use at the patient's bedside:

Duplicate tracheostomy tube

Sterile tracheal dilators

Sterile suction catheters

Suction apparatus

Containers for used equipment

In addition the patient should have a bell, pencil and notepad.

Where a cuffed tracheostomy tube has been used a sterile
10 ml syringe and 1 pair Spencer Wells forceps are required.

The inner tube is changed as required. The one just removed
is cleansed by a sodium bicarbonate solution before being
sterilized ready for further use. Should the tube be dislodged
the nurse must maintain the airway by using the tracheal
dilators until the tube is replaced.

Daily dressing   The dressing of the wound is essentially
the same as for any other wound, but gauze rather than wool
mops should be used. Care should be taken to see that there
are no loose threads which could become detached from the
gauze and harm the patient. Normal saline is usually used for
cleansing the wound. The gauze swabs should be well wrung
out in order to prevent any liquid trickling into the trachea
from around the tracheostomy tube.

After cleansing, a thin fold of gauze is placed between the
skin and the shield of the tracheostomy tube. Tulle gras is
often placed around the opening for the first two or three
days after operation. Clean, sterile tape, is used when necessary to replace that holding the outer tube in position.

The patient with a permanent tracheostomy usually cleanses
the area around the opening himself, using clean, rather than
sterile, equipment. If the skin becomes sore a little cream
may be applied. A thin fold of gauze is cut to the shape of
a bib to fit around the tracheostomy beneath the shield of
the tube.

Lumbar Puncture

Lumbar puncture is performed in order to obtain a specimen
of the cerebrospinal fluid, to estimate the pressure of the fluid,
or to inject drugs intrathecally for diagnosis or treatment. Two
examples of drugs which may be given by this route are

antibiotics, such as streptomycin in the treatment of menin-
gitis, and Myodil, a radio-opaque substance which may be
injected before an X-ray examination of the spinal cord in
cases of injury or suspected new growth. The basic equipment
as previously described on pages 17–18 will be needed. Three
sterile containers for specimens of cerebrospinal fluid should
be provided.

The following sterile equipment is added on the trolley:

Top shelf
    Pack or box containing a glass manometer
    Adaptor and about 10 cm of rubber or polythene tubing
    Lumbar puncture needles
    A two-way tap will be needed unless this is incorporated in
the lumbar puncture needle
    A sterile pack of gloves may be needed.
    Where an antibiotic drug or radio-opaque medium is to be
injected sterile 10 ml and 20 ml syringes will be required; also
the ampoules containing the drug.

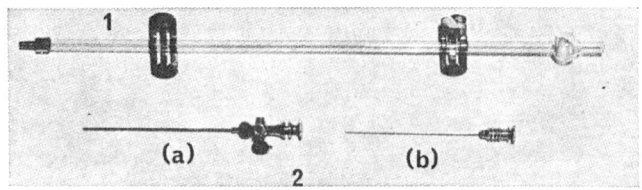

FIG. 10.

1. Manometer   2. Lumbar puncture needles

Position of the Patient

The usual position is left lateral with the patient's chin and
knees as nearly touching as possible and his back along the
edge of the bed. Following the procedure the patient should

rest in bed, lying flat with one pillow under his head for about
six to twelve hours, unless other instructions are given by the
medical staff.

Tapping the Abdomen (Paracentesis Abdominis)

Tapping the abdomen is carried out for the purpose of draining ascitic fluid from the peritoneal cavity. The cause of
the ascites may be congestive cardiac failure, obstruction
of the portal circulation—as in cirrhosis of the liver—the
nephrotic syndrome, or secondary malignant deposits in the
peritoneum.

In addition to the basic equipment listed on pages 17–18
the following sterile equipment will be needed:

Top shelf
Large ascites trocar and cannula
Southey's tubes with shield
Rubber or polythene tubing to fit the cannula to be used
and long enough to reach the drainage receiver
Screw clip
Drip connector may be required: if this is used then 2
separate lengths of tubing should be provided in place of the
one long piece.

Bottom shelf
Container for the drained fluid, e.g. a sterile Winchester
bottle or a 2000 ml plastic drainage bag
Specimen containers, i.e. 2 small sterile bottles for samples
of the fluid
A many-tailed abdominal bandage or a binder.

NOTE: The patient's bladder must be empty before the trocar
and cannula are inserted and a separate trolley for catheterization (*see* p. 62) may be needed.

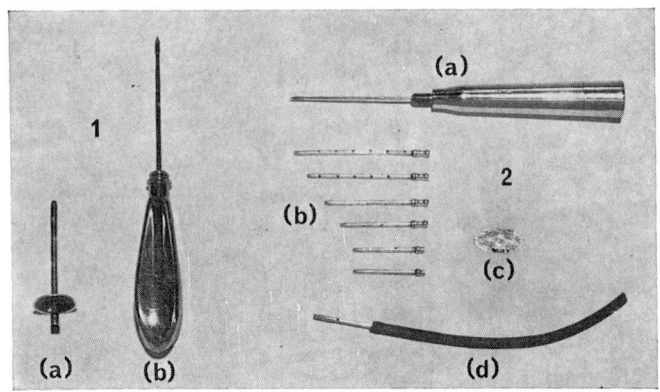

FIG. 11.

1. Large trocar (b); and cannula (a)
2. Southey's tubes: (a) introducer; (b) tubes (tubes usually stored in handle area when not in use); (c) shield; and (d) tube with rubber tubing attached

Position of the Patient

The best position for this procedure, and the one which the patient will usually find most comfortable, is sitting-up and well supported by a back-rest and pillows. The abdominal bandage should be placed in position, but not fastened, before the trocar and cannula are inserted. The usual site for the insertion is in the midline between the umbilicus and the symphysis pubis.

If the fluid drains quickly then the intra-abdominal pressure is rapidly reduced and the patient may suffer from shock. The abdominal bandage must be firmly applied and then tightened from time to time as the fluid drains in order to maintain the intra-abdominal pressure.

Tapping the Legs

Tapping the legs to remove oedematous fluid may be used to relieve gross oedema in congestive cardaic failure or the nephrotic syndrome (subacute glomerulonephritis).

Southey's tubes without the shield (usually four of the smallest size) are used.

Sterile drainage containers may be needed. Alternatively the fluid may drain into large sterile dressings which will need changing at frequent intervals.

Peritoneal Dialysis

Peritoneal dialysis is an alternative to the 'artificial kidney' method of removing end-products of protein breakdown and other toxic materials from the blood of the anuric patient whose kidneys are unable to excrete these substances.

In each method the underlying principle is the exchange of substances in solution through a semipermeable membrane. In the artificial kidney the process used is haemodialysis and involves removing the patient's blood via an arterial catheter and allowing it to flow in a thin film along one side of a cellophane membrane, on the other side of which is the dialysing fluid. The toxic substances in the blood are exchanged with the electrolytes in the dialysing solution and the detoxicated blood is returned to one of the patient's peripheral veins.

Peritoneal dialysis uses the patient's own peritoneum as the dialysing membrane and the dialysing fluid is introduced via a special catheter inserted into the peritoneal cavity and then siphoned out. If necessary, electrolyte imbalance can be corrected by adding the required electrolytes to the isotonic dialysing fluid. Heparin may be added to prevent fibrin formation and an antibiotic, such as tetracycline, added as a bacteriostatic.

Peritoneal dialysis is simpler and less costly than the artificial kidney and it does not necessitate the removal of the patient to a special unit. Some of the indications for dialysis are acute and chronic renal failure, acute circulatory failure, poisoning, as for example from barbiturates and Aspirin.

In addition to the equipment for special investigations and treatment as listed on pages 17–18, omitting specimen containers and pathological request forms, the following equipment is required:

Top shelf

Skin sutures, e.g. black thread size 2/0

Sterile half-circle cutting edge needles

Sterile needle-holder

Packs containing sterile dialysis equipment and dialysis catheter.

Bottom shelf

Pack (or bottle) of sterile dialysing solution, e.g. Dianeal solution

Sterile graduated drainage bag or bottle and sterile tubing to connect this to the Y-connector of the dialysing set

Heparin, if required

Antibiotic, as ordered

Local anaesthetic, e.g. lignocaine 1% solution

Fluid balance record.

Care of the Patient

After the treatment has begun, regular observations of the patient's temperature, pulse and respiration should be made during the period of dialysis; for example, the physician may require these observations to be made at hourly, or half-hourly intervals. Any evidence of shock, abdominal distension or bleeding should be reported at once. Should the patient become restless or complain of pain the doctor should be informed.

If the draining is inadequate and the simple measures of

changing the patient's position or applying slight, brief pressure over the lower abdomen fail, then the doctor may need to change the catheter.

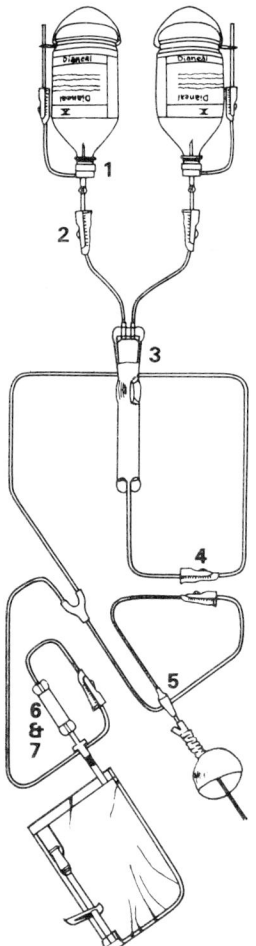

Fig. 12. Peritoneal dialysis administration set

1. Connectors with integral airways fit all types of solution containers

2. 'Flo-trol' clamps facilitate bottle changes

3. Filter and drip chamber

4. 'Flo-trol' clamps for administration and drainage control

5. 'Flashball' injection site for supplemental medication

6. Back stop chamber on drainage tubing

7. Drainage bag connector

Aspiration of the Pleural Cavity

X-ray examination is carried out to determine the presence
and site of a pleural effusion. Following this, the fluid may be
removed by aspiration. A pleural effusion may be due to
inflammation, as in pneumonia or pulmonary tuberculosis, or
it may be a non-inflammatory transudate as in the generalized
oedema of congestive cardiac failure or the nephrotic syndrome. Pleural effusion may also occur in malignant disease
of the lung and following chest injury.

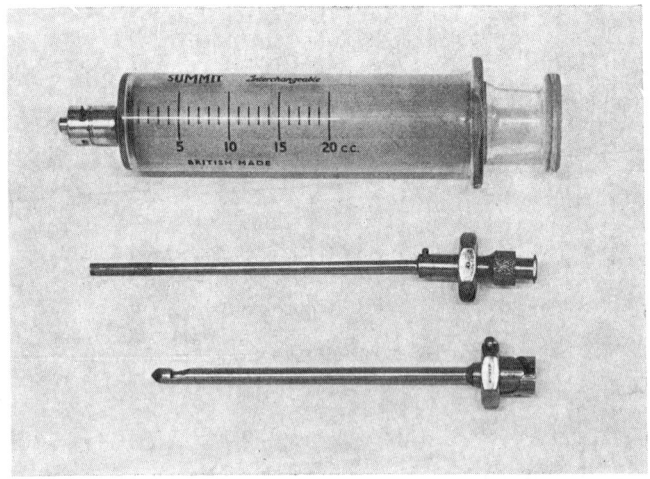

FIG. 13. Luer-Lok syringe; and Abram's pleural biopsy needles

In addition to the basic equipment listed on pages 17–18
the following sterile equipment will be needed:

Top shelf

20 ml syringe with a locking device to provide an airtight
connection with a chest aspiration needle. Martin's syringe or
a Luer-Lok syringe may be used

Selection of aspirating needles

A two-way tap

Rubber or polythene tubing to fit the tap, approximately 15 cm long

Sterile measure jug of 1000 ml capacity.

Bottom shelf

Specimen containers, 2 sterile bottles.

NOTE: The patient's chest X-rays and a viewing box should also be available.

Position of the Patient

The patient is required to sit up and lean forward. If he is in bed he leans forward resting his arms on a pillow supported on a bed table in front of him. The other pillows are removed except for one which may be left supporting the lower part of his back. The patient should be sufficiently far down the bed to allow enough space between him and the bed-head for easy access to the posterior chest wall.

If the patient is not confined to bed he can sit astride a chair with his arms folded and resting on the back of the chair.

A linctus may be prescribed to reduce coughing.

Following the procedure the patient should rest in whatever position he finds most comfortable. Any sudden increase in respiration rate, or complaint of pain in the chest, should be reported immediately.

Underwater Seal Drain

In the normal way, there is a negative pressure in the pleural space between the lung and the chest wall. If, because of injury, the wall of this space is punctured then either air or fluid may enter causing collapse of the lung and ultimate impairment of lung function.

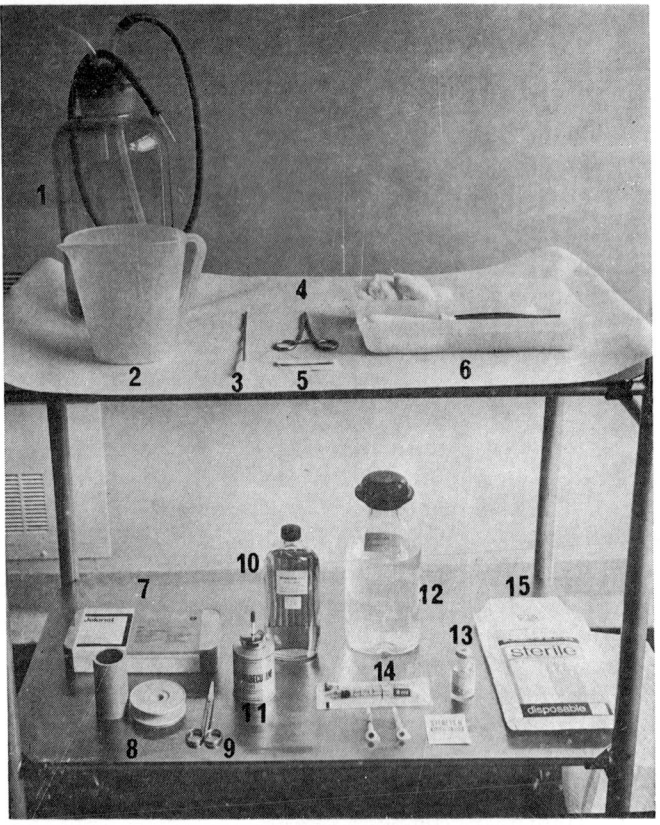

Fig. 14. Underwater seal drain

1. Tudor Edward's bottle, tubing and connection
2. Sterile measure jug
3. Trocar and catheter
4. Needle-holding forceps
5. Black thread with cutting needle
6. Dressing equipment
7. 'Jelonet'
8. Strapping
9. Scissors
10. Skin cleansing lotion
11. Plastic spray dressing
12. Sterile water
13. Local anaesthetic
14. Syringe and needles
15. Sterile gloves

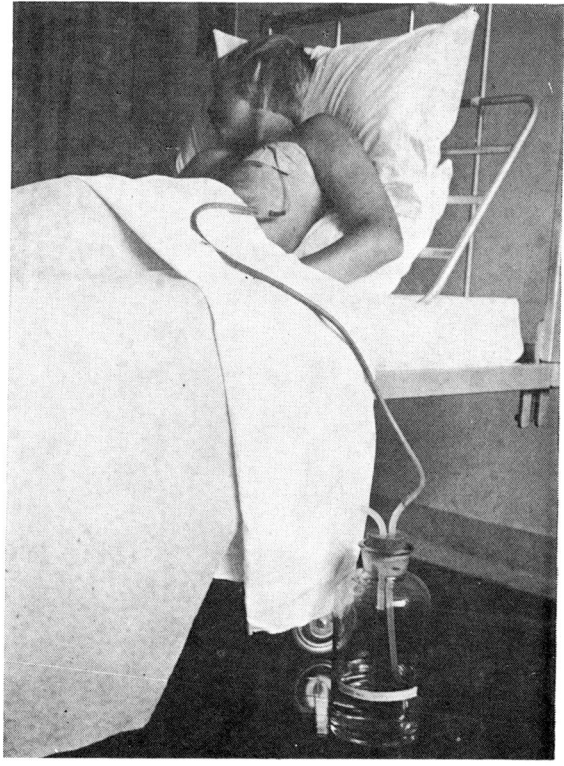

FIG. 15. Underwater seal drain *in situ*

It may therefore become urgently necessary to insert an underwater seal drain to remove the collection of air or fluid and therefore allow full re-expansion of the lung.

In addition to the basic equipment listed on pages 17–18, the following items will be needed:

Top shelf
   Tudor Edwards bottle and tubing
   Connection
   Sterile measure jug
   Black thread with cutting needle
   Needle-holding forceps
   Trocar and catheter.

Bottom shelf
   Sterile water (1 l)
   'Jelonet'
   Local anaesthetic
   Syringe and needles
   Plastic spray dressing
   Waterproof strapping
   Sterile gloves
   Suction apparatus may be required.

As will be realized, the nursing care of a patient who has had an underwater seal drain inserted is very specialized and a nurse should have received specific instruction and understand the rules for the care of the underwater seal drain to ensure its continued efficient functioning.

Pleural Biopsy

Pleural biopsy, which involves obtaining a small piece of parietal pleura, is usually undertaken to determine whether a pleural effusion is of tuberculous or malignant origin.
   The following sterile equipment should be added on the trolley of equipment for pleural aspiration:

Top shelf
   Pleural biopsy needle
   Two-way tap to fit syringe and needles
   Small cutting edge skin needle and skin suture.

Position of the Patient

The position of the patient is the same as that described for pleural aspiration.

Following the investigation the patient should remain in bed for twenty-four hours, during which time regular observation of the pulse and respirations should be made. As a general rule, the patient does not experience any severe pain or discomfort following this procedure but changes in pulse or respiration rates, complaint of pain in the chest or any deterioration in his condition should be reported immediately.

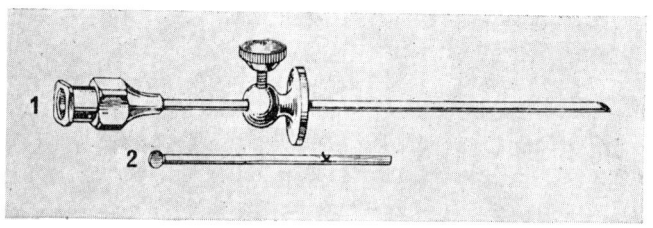

FIG. 16.

1. Menghini liver biopsy needle   2. Nail contained in needle shaft

Liver Biopsy

Liver biopsy is used as an aid to diagnosis in suspected chronic disease of the liver. The sample of tissue is obtained by puncturing the liver with a special needle. Before the biopsy the patient's blood is grouped and cross-matched and the haemoglobin and prothrombin content, the clotting and bleeding times are estimated. The biopsy is not usually carried out if the prothrombin content is found to be below 70 % of the normal.

In addition to the basic equipment as listed on pages 17–18 the following sterile equipment is required:

Top shelf
    Liver biopsy needle, e.g. Menghini's needle (this can be obtained in disposable form)
    10 ml and 20 ml syringes.

Bottom shelf
    Specimen containers—2 bottles containing formaldehyde in normal saline.

Position of the Patient

The patient should be lying on his back as near the right-hand edge of the bed as possible. His right arm is supported above his head to provide clear access to the right intercostal spaces. The needle is introduced in the mid-or the anterior, axillary line between the eighth and ninth, or the ninth and tenth ribs.

    Following the investigation the patient should rest in bed for twenty-four hours during which time regular observations of the pulse and blood pressure should be made. There is a risk of haemorrhage and any rise in pulse rate, fall in blood pressure, complaint of pain or any other signs of deterioration in the patient's condition should be reported at once.

Marrow Biopsy (Bone Marrow Puncture)

Marrow biopsy is carried out as a diagnostic procedure in suspected cases of leukaemia, aplastic anaemia, multiple myeloma and a number of other conditions affecting the blood cells.

    The following sterile equipment should be added to the basic equipment listed on pages 17–18.

Top shelf
    Marrow puncture needle
    10 ml or 20 ml syringe.

Bottom shelf

Glass slides for the specimens of bone marrow and methyl alcohol for fixing the smears will be needed.

Position of the Patient

The patient usually lies flat with his head resting on one pillow. The marrow specimen may be aspirated from the sternum or from the iliac crest.

The patient may be given a sedative beforehand and after the investigation he should be allowed to rest in any comfortable position.

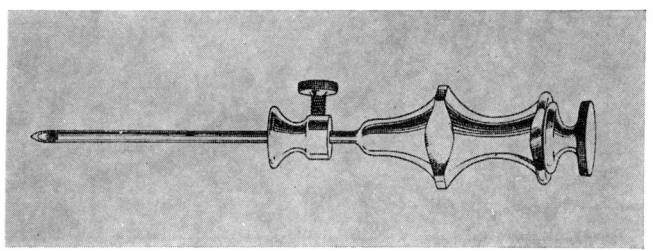

FIG. 17. Needle for sternal puncture for marrow biopsy

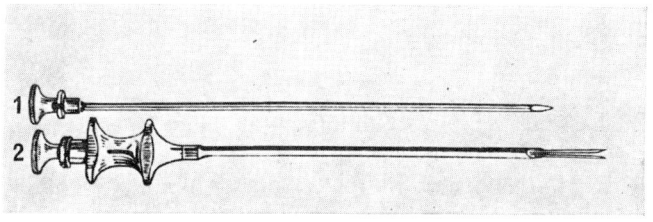

FIG. 18. Vim Silverman's renal biopsy needle:

1. Short cannula   2. Needle with split cannula in
                                        position

Renal Biopsy

Renal biopsy is one of the measures which may be needed in the investigation of renal disease, and is usually carried out under X-ray control. The results of previous investigation such as X-ray examination, renal function tests and the blood clotting time should be collected ready for the doctor who is carrying out the biopsy. Immediately before the procedure the patient should empty his bladder.

In addition to the basic equipment as listed on pages 17–18, the following sterile equipment should be added:

Top shelf
Renal biopsy needle, e.g. Vim-Silverman's needle
2 10 ml syringes
Gloves.

Bottom shelf
Specimen containers—2 bottles containing formaldehyde in normal saline
Crepe pressure bandage.

Position of the Patient

The patient should lie prone on a hard surface which the X-ray table provides. A sandbag must be provided which the doctor will usually put in position under the patient's abdomen in order to fix the kidney against the dorsal surface of the body.

Following the investigation, a pressure bandage should be applied and the patient should be kept at rest in bed for twenty-four hours and for the first twelve hours he should lie flat with his head resting on one pillow. Regular observations of the pulse and blood pressure should be made and a rise in pulse rate or fall in blood pressure, pain or any other sign of deterioration in the patient's condition should be reported at once. The wound should be inspected at regular intervals. Haematuria is common after this procedure. It is usually slight but should be reported immediately. Urine passed during the first twenty-four hours may be required for inspection; each specimen is labelled with the date and the time at which it was passed. The patient should be encouraged to take frequent fluids.

Intestinal (Jejunal) Biopsy

Intestinal biopsy in order to obtain a specimen of the jejunal mucosa is one of several investigations that may be needed in the diagnosis of the malabsorption condition known as the coeliac syndrome. A small metal capsule (Crosby's capsule) attached to a long fine tube is passed via the nose or mouth into the jejunum. The position of the capsule is confirmed by X-ray.

The following equipment is required:

Top shelf
    Crosby's capsule and tube
    20 ml syringe.

Bottom shelf
    Bottle containing normal saline
    3 specimen bottles
    Roger's throat spray
    Lignocaine 4% solution

NOTE: If the tube is not radio-opaque then an opaque medium, e.g. gastrographin, and a syringe to introduce this into the Crosby tube will be needed.

    Receiver for the capsule after use
    Vomit bowl and paper tissues should be at hand in case the patient vomits.

NOTE: As no puncture is made in the skin surface for the procedure, the dressing instruments, knife blades and handles and other equipment described under 'basic requirements' will not be needed. The local anaesthetic is applied by spray and therefore the syringe and needles for local infiltration will not be required.

Care of the Patient

Following the investigation the patient should rest in bed for twenty-four hours. Regular observations of the pulse should be made and the stools saved and examined for evidence of bleeding.

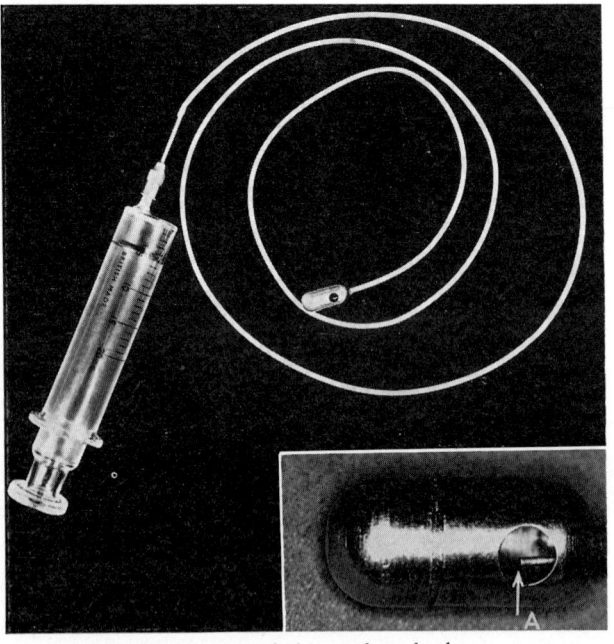

FIG. 19. Crosby's capsule and tube

4 Parenteral Administration of Fluids

The term 'parenteral' means outside the alimentary tract and is used to describe the administration of fluids by any route other than by mouth or rectally. The route most frequently used is the venous circulation and intravenous therapy includes the introduction into the circulation of fluids to correct water and electrolyte imbalance and also the administration of blood and plasma, or plasma substitutes. Fluids can be introduced into the peritoneal cavity and normal saline or saline–glucose solution can be given into the subcutaneous tissues.

Intravenous Infusion

Intravenous infusion of fluid is the quickest and most controlled method of replacing serious loss of water and correcting electrolyte imbalance. The fluid to be given will depend on the condition which requires treatment. Examples of replacement fluids are:

1. Normal saline solution: 9 g sodium chloride per litre of water, providing sodium and water.
2. Dextrose solution: 50 g dextrose per litre, providing water and some calories.
3. Sodium lactate ($\frac{1}{6}$ molar solution) for alkali replacement.
4. Hartman or Darrow or Butler's solutions, which replace loss of cellular electrolytes and contain potassium. Accurate measurement and recording of all fluid intake and output must be maintained whenever intravenous therapy is employed.

In addition to the basic equipment as listed on pages 17–18, but omitting specimen containers and pathology request forms, the following equipment is required:

Bottom shelf

Bottle or plastic container of the sterile fluid to be given

Pack containing sterile 'giving' set. These packs are usually obtained ready for use from a commercial firm, and contain the following: (a) the 'giving' needle; (b) a length of polythene tubing; (c) a drip chamber (also known as a drop counter); (d) a needle to perforate the seal of the container, and (e) a screw clip

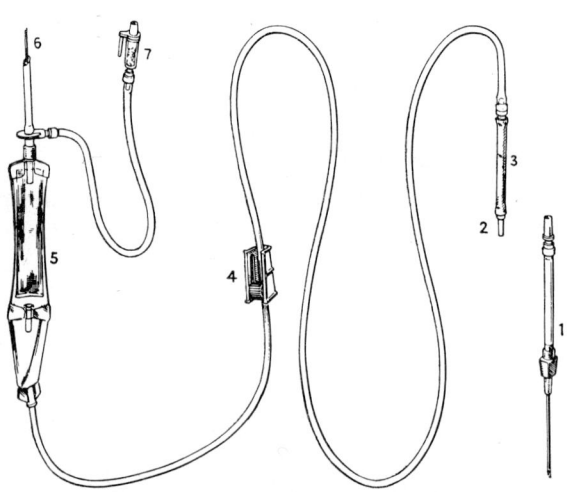

FIG. 20. Disposable polythene 'giving set'

1. Intravenous needle
2. and 3. Luer fitting mount attached to polythene tubing
4. Clamp
5. Combined nylon filter and drop counter
6. Perforating needle
7. Air inlet filter to be hooked above the fluid level in the container

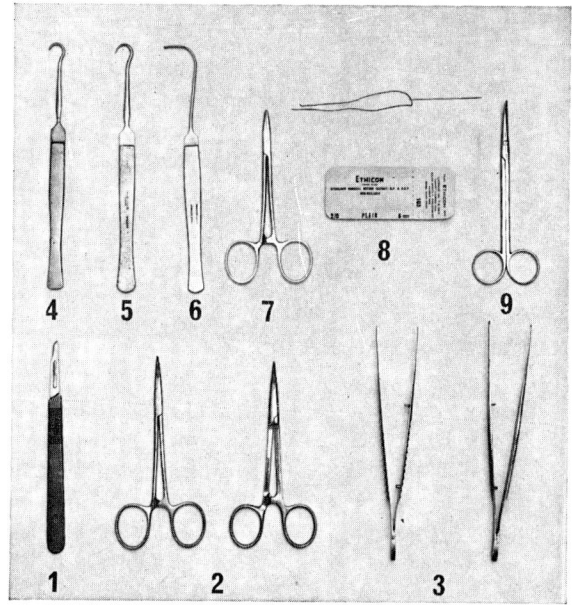

FIG. 21. Instruments for exposure of a vein

1. Bard-Parker blade and handle
2. Fine artery forceps
3. Dissecting forceps
4. Blunt hook
5. Sharp hook
6. Aneurysm needle
7. Needle-holder
8. Suture materials
9. Fine stitch scissors

Sphygmomanometer

Waterproof square

Waterproof cover for the pillow

Straight splint for the limb into which the infusion is to be given (if required)

Crepe or 'Kling' bandage

Razor and blade for shaving site

A transfusion stand will be needed if this is not incorporated in the bedstead frame.

Exposing a vein   In some cases where an intravenous infusion is needed it may be necessary to expose a vein and introduce a cannula. The nurse may often hear this procedure described colloquially as a 'cut down'. The following equipment should be added:

Top shelf

Instrument dish or a pack containing:

2 pairs toothed dissecting forceps

2 pairs fine ('mosquito') artery forceps

1 blunt hook

1 sharp hook

1 aneurysm needle

1 pair fine stitch scissors

Suture materials, e.g. catgut size oo, thread size oo and 2 fine cutting edge skin needles

1 needle-holder

Intravenous cannula or fine polythene tubing and an adaptor.

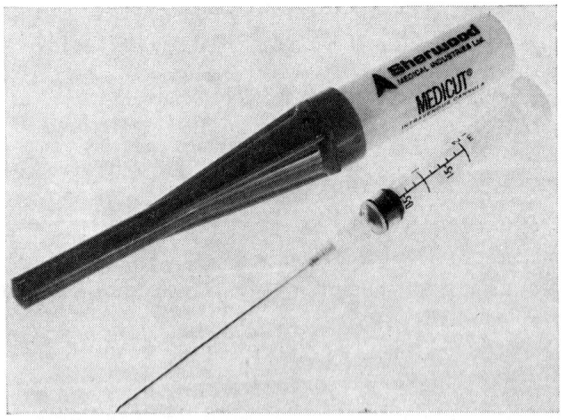

FIG. 22. Disposable intravenous cannula

Transfusion of Blood and Plasma

Transfusion of blood or plasma is required in the treatment of shock accompanying injury, such as crushing injuries and major fractures, burns, and serious loss of blood from any cause including major surgery. Transfusion fluids available are:

1. Whole blood.
2. Concentrated suspension of red cells.
3. Dried plasma with sterile pyrogen-free water for reconstitution (less commonly used).
4. Plasma substitute, e.g. 6% dextran solution.

Before a blood transfusion is started a careful check is made to ensure that the right blood is given to the right patient. The container is labelled showing the ABO and RH groups, the expiry date of the blood, the patient's name, hospital number and ward and the statement that the direct cross-matching tests show that the blood in the container and the patient's blood are compatible. The particulars on the label are checked with the patient's prescription sheet and identity band.

Blood containers must be handled carefully to avoid shaking the contents. Stored blood is kept at a temperature between 4°C and 6°C (39-43°F). Blood must not be warmed.

The basic equipment required is as described for intravenous infusion. The container of blood is placed on the bottom shelf of the trolley and a bottle of sterile normal saline solution may also be needed. The disposable 'giving set' selected must be one with a filter incorporated. A number of different sets have been designed for special needs—for example, for giving blood or other fluids under pressure and for intravenous therapy for young children. In such cases the nurse should ascertain the particular set required. Instructions for use of sterile disposable sets of all types are usually clearly set out on the cover of the pack.

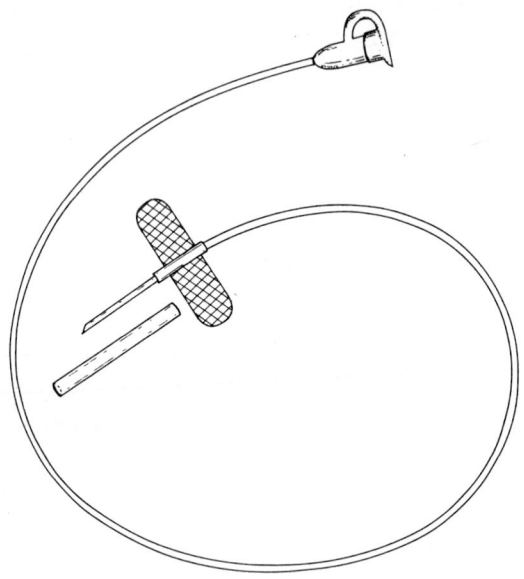

FIG. 23. Scalp vein needle used in paediatric intravenous therapy

Subcutaneous Infusion

Subcutaneous infusion as a method of giving fluid is more often used for young children and infants than for adults. The solution used may be normal saline, or 0·5 % saline (sodium chloride) solution with or without the addition of 2·5 % glucose. Stronger glucose solutions are liable to cause tissue necrosis. Sites for injection are the outer aspects of the thighs,

the anterior axillary areas and the anterior chest wall below
the breasts.

Drip infusions are given into two sites simultaneously.

In addition to the basic equipment as described on pages
17–18, the following sterile equipment is required:

Top shelf

An instrument dish, or packs, containing:

2 needles for subcutaneous infusion (No. 17 or 20 gauge)
6–7·5 cm long, and adaptors

Y-shaped connection

2 lengths of tubing each about 30 cm long to fit the adaptor, or if adaptors are not used, to fit the hub of the needle, and
the arms of a Y-shaped connector

Length of tubing to fit the single arm of the Y-shaped
connector and the drip chamber

About 15 cm of tubing to connect the drip chamber to the
outlet tube of the bottle containing the infusion fluid.

Bottom shelf

Bottle of sterile solution for the infusion.

NOTE: A subcutaneous infusion may, in the case of infants, be
given as a single slow injection using a 20 ml syringe and
needle.

Intraperitoneal Infusion

Intraperitoneal infusion can be a useful method of introducing fluid in the treatment of dehydration in infants where
the small size of the veins can make intravenous therapy
difficult, and when fluid is required more urgently than can
be given by subcutaneous infusion.

The solution used may be normal saline or glucose–saline
and quantities of up to 300 ml can be given quite quickly,

i.e. in fifteen to thirty minutes. The site for the insertion of the needle is the lower part of the abdomen, a little below the umbilicus and to one side of the midline.

Equipment needed is as for intravenous infusion omitting the sphygmomanometer, straight splint and bandage.

5 Parenteral Administration of Drugs

The term 'parenteral' (outside the alimentary tract) in relation to the administration of drugs, includes subcutaneous (hypodermic), intramuscular and intravenous injections.

Many of the drugs commonly given by injection are potentially toxic substances which come under the control of the Poisons and Pharmacy Act and also, if they are drugs liable to lead to addiction, the Controlled Drugs Act. Regulations made under these Acts control the ordering of stocks, the storing and the prescribing of such drugs. In addition, the hospital usually lays down rules for the checking, administration, and recording of all drugs given by injection. The main points covered are:

1. The prescription must be carefully read and checked by the person witnessing and the person giving the drug.

2. When the drug is obtained from the cupboard it is checked with the prescription.

3. The prescribed dose is drawn up into the syringe in the presence of the witness who checks the calculation (if any), the measured dose and the name of the patient.

4. The injection is taken to the bedside, the identity of the patient is checked again and the medication is then given in the presence of the witness.

5. The patient's name, the hospital number, the drug, the dose, the date and time of its administration, are entered in the ward record and signed in full by the person giving the injection and the person witnessing it.

A tray containing the following equipment is required:

1. Sterile syringe and needle of suitable size for the particular injection.

NOTE: In some hospitals sterile disposable syringes and needles are used, in others reusable syringes and needles are provided, sterilized by dry heat in metal containers. Where there is no central supply, the usual method of sterilizing is by boiling and the syringe and needle are then dished into a sterile tray and may be stored in spirit or in instrument solution. In such cases the syringe and needle must be rinsed in sterile water before use. If record type syringes are used the metal plunger and the glass barrel must be separated before boiling, otherwise the rapid expansion of the metal will break the glass.

2. Sterile swabs and lotion for cleaning the skin, e.g. a packet containing swabs impregnated with surgical spirit or a container with sterile wool mops and gallipot, or a spray bottle, with an antiseptic solution.

3. The patient's prescription sheet.

4. The prescribed drug. If the drug is dispensed in a glass ampoule, a piece of gauze will be needed to break the neck of the ampoule.

Subcutaneous (Hypodermic) Injection

Select a 1 ml or 2 ml syringe according to the quantity to be injected and a needle of suitable size.

Subcutaneous injection is commonly used for the administration of drugs which are non-irritating to the superficial tissues and require only a small quantity of fluid to be injected. Examples of drugs given by this method are insulin and adrenaline. The usual sites for injection are the outer aspect of the upper arm and the front of the thigh.

Intramuscular Injection

The three sites for intramuscular injection are:

1. The middle third aspect of the thigh. To give an injection (a) of large volume and (b) irritant substances into the thigh, proceed thus. Using both hands, place the middle finger of one hand on the femoral epicondyle below, and the middle finger of the other hand on the greater trochanter above, then using thumbs and hand span, divide the femur into thirds, and give the injection into the outer side (antero-lateral aspect) of the middle third of the thigh as shown in the diagram.

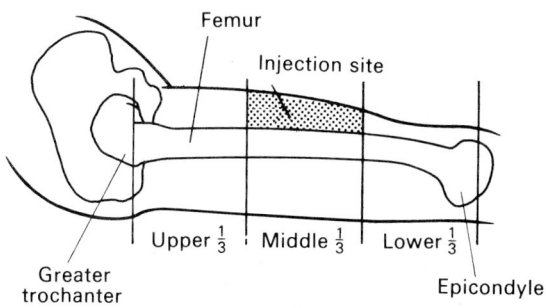

FIG. 24. Intramuscular injection site: middle third aspect of thigh

2. Outer aspect of the shoulder. Small 2 ml injections can be given into the deltoid muscle on the outer aspect of the shoulder. The shoulder should be exposed, so that the site may be accurately determined.

3. Upper and outer quadrant of the buttock. For an intramuscular injection of large volume to be given into the buttock, place the patient in lateral position, divide the area in

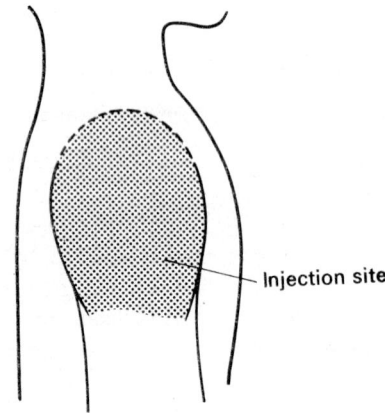

FIG. 25. Intramuscular injection site: outer aspect of shoulder

half by drawing an imaginary horizontal line and a vertical line from the greater trochanter of the femur to the natal cleft. The injection is given into the upper, outer quadrant (quarter), as is indicated by the shaded area on the diagram. The illustration also shows the relevant position of the under-lying structures.

Drugs injected into muscle are more rapidly absorbed than those injected into subcutaneous tissue. This is because muscle is very well supplied with blood. There is less risk of local irritation and larger amounts can be injected than can com-fortably be given by subcutaneous injection. Examples of drugs given by intramuscular injection are antibiotics, vita-mins and iron preparations.

Since the needle must penetrate deeply into the tissues there is a risk of puncturing a blood vessel or a nerve unless proper precautions are taken. In order to avoid giving the injection into a vein, the plunger of the syringe is withdrawn slightly after the needle has been inserted and if blood appears in the

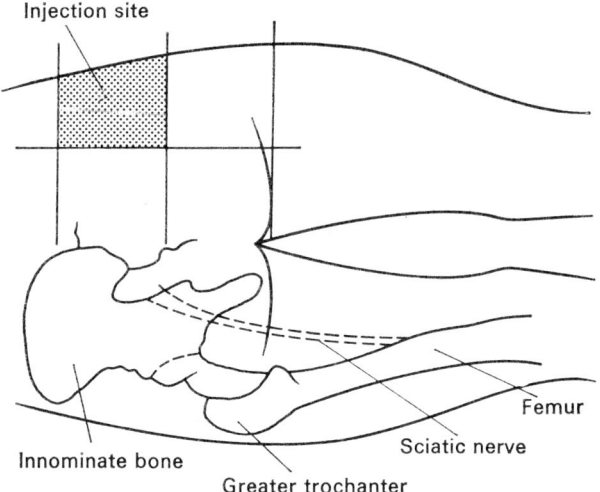

Injection site

Femur

Sciatic nerve

Innominate bone

Greater trochanter

FIG. 26. Intramuscular injection site: upper and outer quadrant of the buttock

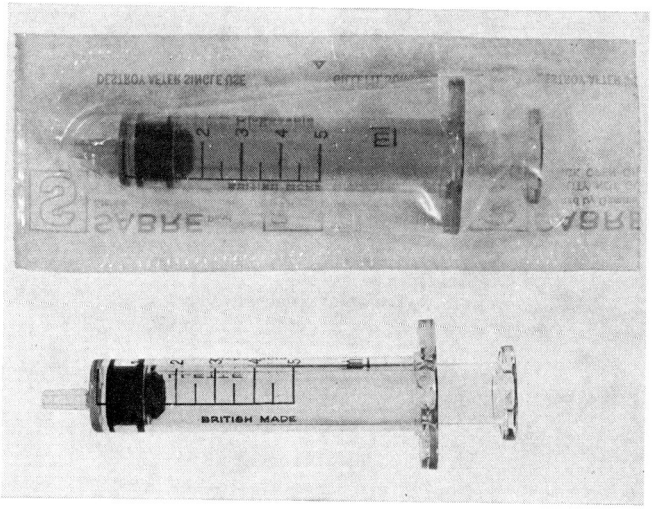

FIG. 27. Sterile disposable syringe

syringe the position of the needle must be changed slightly. If no blood appears when the plunger is again withdrawn a little, then it is safe to give the injection.

Intravenous Injection

Select a 5 ml or 10 ml syringe according to the amount of fluid to be injected, and a needle of suitable size.

A sterile dressing, such as a small piece of gauze incorporated in a strip of adhesive plaster, may be required to seal the puncture. Oozing of blood when the needle is removed can be stopped by firm pressure with a small pad of sterile gauze.

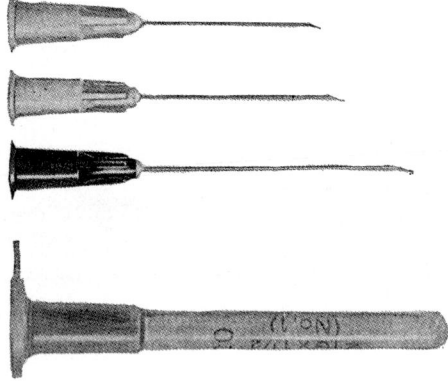

FIG. 28. Sterile disposable needles

A length of rubber tubing or a sphygmomanometer, to act as a tourniquet and make the veins more prominent is required if one of the veins on the anterior aspect of elbow (median cephalic or median basilic vein) is to be used. Other sites for intravenous injections are the superficial veins on the back of the hand or the leg just above the ankle (the short saphenous vein and its tributaries). For infants and young children the superficial veins of the neck or the scalp may be chosen. Intravenous injection of drugs is, with rare exceptions, a procedure which is carried out by a member of the medical staff. Drugs introduced directly into the circulation have an immediate action and therefore the effect of the medication is much greater than that of an equivalent dose given intramuscularly, or subcutaneously, and more slowly absorbed.

Where an intravenous infusion is already in progress, prescribed drugs may be introduced via a three-way tap or through a specially designed area of the tubing of the 'giving' set which has self-sealing qualities.

Drugs to be used in this way are usually given by a doctor or a trained nurse, depending upon hospital policy.

Examples of drugs given intravenously because rapid action is needed are bronchodilators and anaesthetic agents.

Drugs may be given intravenously for diagnostic purposes such as the contrast media used in X-ray examinations, e.g. water-soluble iodine compounds used in X-ray examinations such as intravenous pyelography and cholecystography.

If traces of the drug and, particularly after intravenous injection, blood, are allowed to dry in the syringe and needle, effective cleaning is difficult. A bowl of cold disinfectant solution should be at hand in which the used syringe and needle can be placed immediately. This is, of course, not necessary if disposable syringes and needles are used.

6 Vaginal Examination and Treatments

Examination

Vaginal examination may be required for the following reasons:

1. In obstetric practice as part of an antenatal examination; in labour to confirm the onset of labour, to assess the degree of dilation of the cervix uteri and to confirm the position of the foetus.

2. To determine the position of the uterus or the presence, position, and character of a pelvic mass.

3. To inspect the vagina and cervix uteri.

4. To obtain material for bacteriological or cytological examination.

In some cases, such as those mentioned in (2) above, the full set of equipment listed will not be necessary and the few items required, i.e. a vaginal speculum and a pair of examination gloves may be supplied, clean but not sterile. For a full vaginal examination, and particularly if the patient to be examined has undergone vaginal or uterine surgery or has had an abortion, is in labour or is recently delivered, the equipment listed for the top shelf of the trolley must be sterile.

Top shelf
   Pack or bowl containing 2 dressing towels (paper or cloth), wool mops and gauze swabs
   Cusco's bivalve speculum

Sims' speculum
1 pair of sponge-holding forceps
1 pair volsellum forceps
1 uterine sound
2 pairs large artery forceps, e.g. curved and straight

Bottom shelf
Sterile 'throat' swabs
Cervical smear spatulae
Glass slides and cover slips
Bowl or pack containing 2 sanitary towels
Spirit lamp and matches
Pathology request forms
Sterile gloves
0·5 % aqueous chlorhexidine
Paper bag attached to trolley rail or foot-operated pedal bin
at side of trolley for dressings
Paper bag for instruments
Lubricant.

NOTE: If an Anglepoise lamp is not available, add a hand lamp to the bottom shelf. Provision should be made to keep the patient's chest covered and warm during the examination.

Vulval Swabbing

Vulval swabbing, including also the toilet of the perineal area, may be required following operations on the vulva, vagina and perineum, or suture of the perineum following childbirth.

Perineal sutures should be kept dry and usually a piece of gauze is placed around the stitches which must be changed after the use of the bed pan and on each occasion after swabbing.

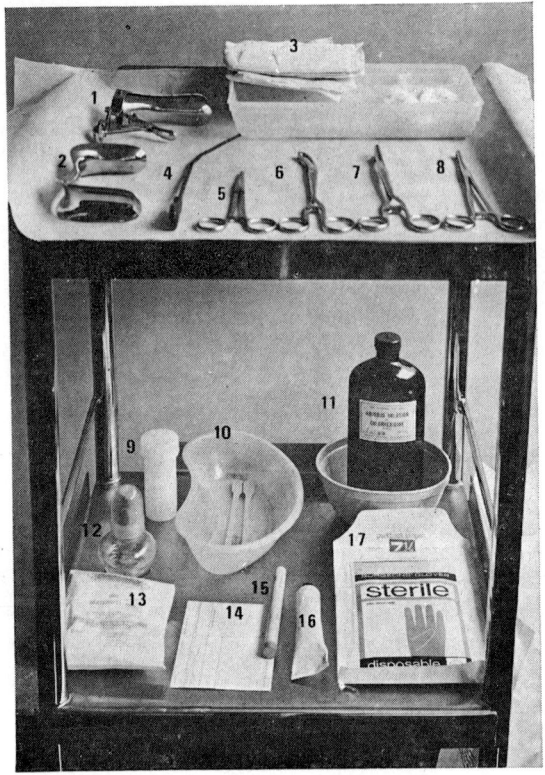

FIG. 29. A vaginal examination trolley

1. Cusco's speculum
2. Sims' speculum
3. Pack or bowl containing 2 dressing towels, wool mops and gauze swabs
4. Uterine sound
5. Straight artery forceps
6. Volsellum forceps
7. Sponge-holding forceps
8. Curved artery forceps
9. Culture slides in container
10. Cervical smear spatulae in receiver
11. 0·5% aqueous chlorhexidine
12. Spirit lamp
13. Sanitary towel
14. Pathological request form
15. Sterile 'throat' swabs
16. Lubricant
17. Sterile gloves

A trolley containing the following basic sterile equipment is required for vulval swabbing and all local treatment:

Bowl or pack of wool mops, gauze and sanitary pad
2 pairs sterile dressing forceps
Bowl of warm lotion—temperature 38-40 °C (100-105 °F) for swabbing, e.g. 0·5 % aqueous chlorhexidine
Paper bag for soiled dressings
Protective square for bed
A bandage or belt to retain the sanitary pad in position.

NOTE: A hand lamp is required if an Anglepoise lamp or other source of adequate lighting is not available.

Vaginal Irrigation (Vaginal Douche)

Vaginal irrigation or douching is now less commonly ordered than in the past but may be required as part of the routine preparation of the patient for vaginal operations or for patients who have a profuse or offensive vaginal discharge.

As a general rule only mild non-irritating lotions are used, such as normal saline. The quantity of lotion required is usually 2 l. The temperature of the lotion for a cleansing douche is 40·5 °C (105 °F). Hot irrigations at a temperature of 46-48 °C (115-118 °F) for the treatment of pelvic inflammation or uterine haemorrhage are now unusually, if ever, employed.

NOTE: Lotion thermometers have not been included in the lists of equipment on the trolley as it has been assumed that solutions will be prepared at the correct strength and temperature in the preparation area.

In addition to the equipment needed for vulval swabbing the following sterile items are required:

Bowl containing:

    Douche can

    Rubber or polythene tubing carrying screw clip

    Douche nozzle, preferably plastic

Jug of prescribed douche lotion at body temperature, e.g. normal saline

    Bed pan.

The colloquial phrase 'jug douche' does not mean a vaginal douche. It is simply an elaboration of vulval swabbing. To equipment for vulval swabbing add a jug of warm cleansing lotion. A bed pan is required.

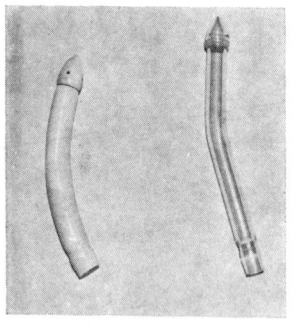

Fig. 30. Douche nozzles: plastic; (left) glass (right)

Insertion of Pessaries

Medicated Pessaries

Medicated pessaries may be ordered for the further treatment of vaginal infections as, for example, nystatin pessaries used in the treatment of monilial infection.

The prescribed pessaries should be added to the equipment for vulval swabbing.

The pessaries may, or may not be supplied with an applicator. If there is no applicator, the following items should be added to the requirements:

Sterile rubber or disposable gloves and glove powder

Tube of obstetric cream

Pack or receiver containing sterile sponge-holding forceps

Cusco's speculum may be required.

Supportive or Corrective Pessaries

Supportive and corrective pessaries are inserted into the vagina to support a prolapsed uterus or to correct retroversion of the uterus. The use of pessaries for the treatment of prolapse is becoming increasingly rare as the majority of patients can be more satisfactorily treated by operation. However, pessaries may be used if the patient is unsuitable for operation or while awaiting operation and the nurse is sometimes required to change the ring pessary used in these cases.

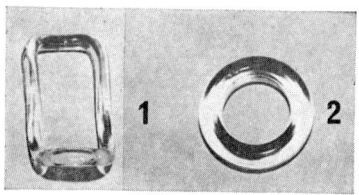

FIG. 31. Supportive and corrective pessaries: 1. Hodge pessary (plastic); 2. ring pessary (plastic)

The type of pessary to be used will be determined by the doctor who also usually inserts it.

In addition to the equipment needed for vulval swabbing, the following items are required:

Sterile packs or receiver containing:
    Sponge-holding forceps
    Pessary to be inserted
    Tube of obstetric cream
Sterile rubber or disposable gloves and glove powder.

NOTE: Where a pessary is to be changed, provide a receptacle for the used pessary when it has been removed.

7 Catheterization and Drainage of the Urinary Bladder

Catheterization

Catheterization of the urinary bladder may be ordered for the following reasons:

1. To empty the bladder in the case of retention of urine occurring as a post-operative complication or as a result of obstruction, as in stricture of the urethra or enlargement of the prostate gland, or where retention is due to disease or injury of the spinal cord.

2. To obtain a specimen of urine from a patient who is unconscious, incontinent, or for any other reason unable to co-operate.

3. To ensure that the bladder is empty before pelvic operations or abdominal paracentesis.

4. After operations on the perineum or vulva to prevent contamination of the operation area. In such cases an indwelling catheter is commonly used.

5. To obtain an uncontaminated specimen of urine for bacteriological examination. Catheterization for this purpose is seldom required for male patients, the collecting of a 'clean' midstream specimen in a sterile container being usually quite satisfactory. In the majority of cases it is usually possible to obtain a 'clean' specimen from a female patient thus avoiding catheterization which always carries some risk of infection.

6. To ensure that urinary output is accurately measured at frequent intervals, to determine renal function.

Catheterization of a Female Patient

The following equipment is required:

Top shelf

Selection of catheters, assorted sizes

Bowl or pack of 2 sterile towels, gauze swabs, wool mops and 2 pairs sterile dissecting forceps

Covered receiver or pack of 2 pairs sterile dissecting forceps

Sterile receiver for urine

Sterile scissors are required if the catheters are in polythene packs, although in many cases the catheters are contained in double packs.

Bottom shelf

Measure jug

Specimen container and pathological examination request form

A bowl of cleansing lotion, e.g. 0·5 % aqueous chlorhexidine

Paper bag for used mops and paper towels

Containers for used instruments and catheters

Protective covering for bed.

NOTE: Where adequate light from an Anglepoise lamp is not available, a hand lamp should be provided. A bed jacket or small blanket should be available to ensure that the patient is kept warm during the procedure.

Self-retaining catheters   Where a self-retaining catheter is to be introduced, the following sterile equipment should be added to inflate the balloon:

Sterile distilled water
1 20 ml syringe
Large bore needle, e.g. No. 2.

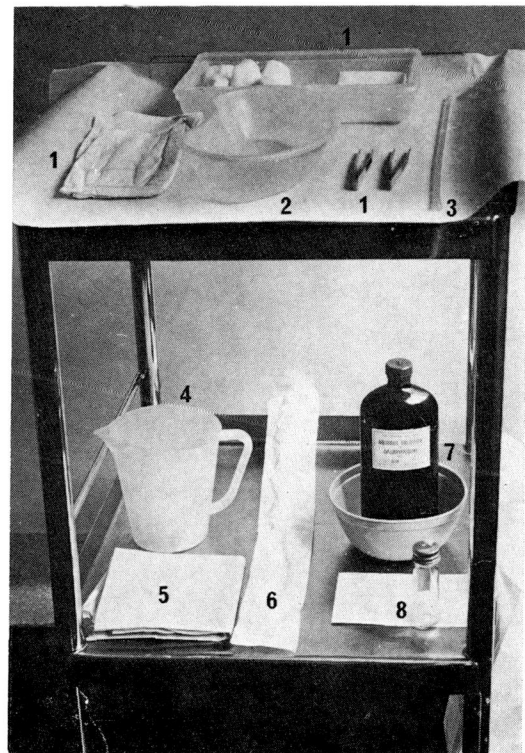

FIG. 32. A trolley showing equipment for catheterization of a female patient

1. Bowl or pack of 2 sterile towels, gauze swabs, wool mops and 2 pairs sterile dissecting forceps
2. Sterile receiver for urine
3. Selected catheter
4. Measure jug
5. Protective covering for bed
6. Reserve catheter
7. 0·5 % aqueous chlorhexidine (in bowl of warm water)
8. Specimen container and pathological examination request form

If intermittent drainage is ordered a sterile spiggot is required.

If continuous drainage is ordered either a sterile Lane's bottle or polythene drainage bag is required. This is connected to the catheter by means of sterile tubing and a straight connector.

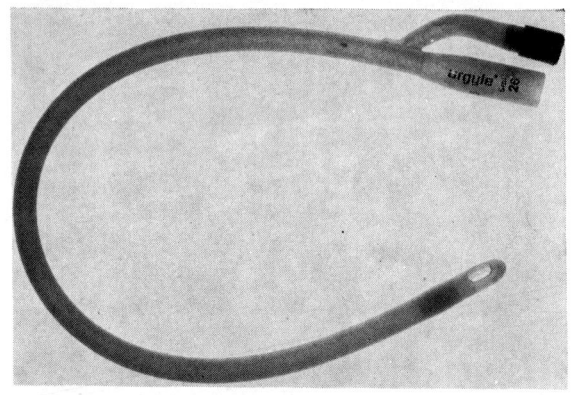

FIG. 33. Argyle's Foley catheter

Catheterization of a Male Patient

The equipment required is basically that for catheterization of a female patient but the following should be added to the trolley:

Urethral applicator
Local anaesthetic, e.g. Xylocaine or Duncaine gel
Lubricant, e.g. sterile glycerine or sterile liquid paraffin.

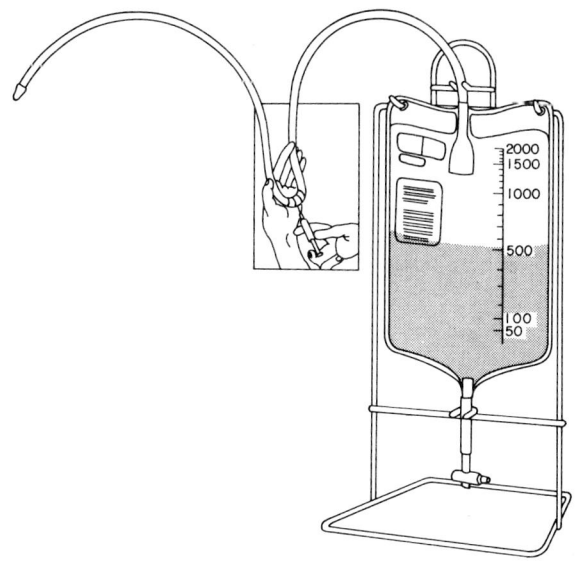

FIG. 34. Disposable drainage bag with drainage tap, urine sampling system and stand

Catheters

Plastic and P.V.C. are the materials commonly used in the production of disposable catheters; they have largely replaced the rubber variety.

Catheters of these materials are more suitable for situations such as obtaining a sterile specimen of urine or for short-term drainage purposes.

Silastic material is also used in the manufacture of catheters but because of the expense involved they are usually reserved for long-term bladder drainage.

The advantage of this material is that it is less irritant to the lining of the urethra and in consequence, there is little formation of stale secretions around the catheter at the urethral meatus.

Catheter Toilet

When a patient has an indwelling catheter there is a serious risk of bladder infection as the catheter provides a pathway for organisms. To prevent possible infection occurring, strict aseptic precautions should be taken whenever the catheter is being released or the tubing and drainage bag changed.

Unless the patient is able to have a daily bath, four-hourly care of the catheter is essential. A tray or trolley containing the following equipment is required:

Bowl or pack of wool mops and gauze
Bowl of warm lotion, e.g. 0·5 % aqueous chlorhexidine
Protective square for bed
Disposal bag for used mops.

Female patients A vulval toilet is carried out, but in addition, the catheter should be cleaned and dried from the urethral meatus downwards.

Male patients The urethral meatus should be cleaned followed by the cleansing of the catheter from above, downwards.

Irrigation of the Bladder

Irrigation of the bladder may be required in conjunction with drainage by an indwelling catheter or, in male patients, to clear the bladder of blood, blood clots and debris following operations.

This procedure is usually ordered for patients who already have a catheter in position. If this is not the case then a trolley for catheterization must be prepared and the equipment listed below for bladder washout added to it:

Top shelf

Jug containing measured quantity (500 ml is usually prepared) of sterile fluid prescribed for washout. The fluid ordered may be normal saline or Hibitane 1 in 5000 solution and should be prepared at body temperature. Washout fluid is available in proprietary sealed containers and should be warmed before use

Large sterile receiver

Sterile bladder syringe (50 ml disposable)

Sterile spigot, or sterile Lane's bottle or drainage bag, if continuous drainage is in progress

A sterile measure jug to hold returned fluid.

NOTE: It is very important to measure the lotion prepared for the washout accurately so that additional drainage may be recorded at the end of the procedure.

8 Rectal Examination, Sigmoidoscopy and Rectal Lavage

Rectal examination by palpation and inspection is often required in such conditions as haemorrhoids, fistula-in-ano and carcinoma of the rectum. It also forms part of the examination of the patient in the investigation of other pelvic conditions such as enlargement of the prostate gland, pelvic abscess, diseases of the uterus and its appendages and appendicitis.

A tray containing the following equipment will be required:

Pairs of rubber or disposable gloves and glove powder
Container of finger cots
Container of gauze and wool mops
Lubricant
Receiver containing proctoscope (battery, leads and spare bulbs if proctoscope is electrically illuminated)
Container for soiled equipment
Paper bag for soiled mops
A hand lamp is required if Anglepoise or other source of adequate light is not available
Equipment for vaginal examination may also be required.

Sigmoidoscopy

Examination of the rectum and sigmoid colon by inspection through an illuminated sigmoidoscope combined with biopsy may be required in the investigation of cases of haemorrhage from the lower part of the bowel and also, when a growth is known to be present, the examination may be carried out in order to obtain information as to its nature, extent and position. Sigmoidoscopy may also be used in the investigation of cases of colitis to assess the condition of the mucous membrane of the bowel.

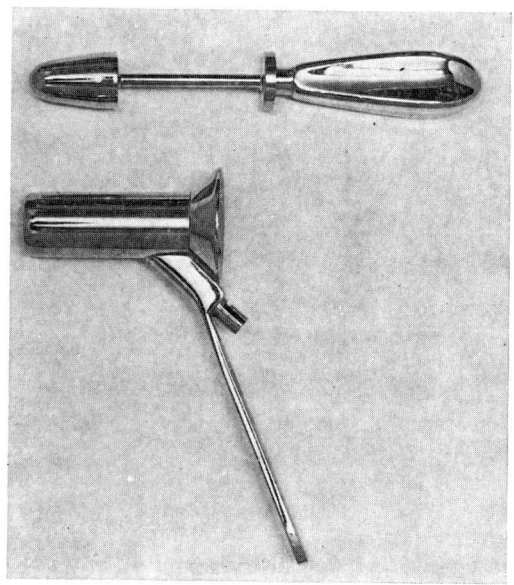

FIG. 35. Proctoscope

The preparation of the patient should begin at least two days beforehand; a light non-residue diet is ordered and an aperient is given. This is followed by an enema or a bisacodyl (Dulcolax) suppository given about twelve hours before the examination. A rectal washout may be ordered to be given four hours before. If the patient is not anaesthetized the sigmoidoscope sheath should be slightly warmed to assist muscular relaxation.

The following equipment is required:

Top shelf
  Pairs of rubber or disposable gloves and glove powder
  Lubricant, e.g. petroleum jelly
  Receiver containing proctoscope and non-tooth dissecting
forceps
  Container of small gauze mops
  Sigmoidoscope, sheath and obturator
  Dissecting forceps
  Biopsy forceps.

Bottom shelf
  Battery, leads, spare bulbs for sigmoidoscope
  Bellows for sigmoidoscope
  Container for used gloves
  Container or paper bag for used mops
  Specimen bottle, labels and pathology request forms
  Protective square for bed
  Suction apparatus may be required.

Rectal Lavage (Washout)

The procedure is carried out to ensure that the lower colon
and rectum are free from faecal matter. This may be necessary
prior to a rectal operation, or the administration of a barium
enema.
  The following equipment is required:

Top shelf
  Bowl containing:
    Catheter (12 EG or 21 FG)
    Rectal tube
    Straight connection
    Tubing, approximately 1 m, carrying screw clip

Funnel

Large jug (5 l capacity) of water or prescribed washout lotion at body temperature

Small jug to carry washout solution to funnel

Lubricant

Container of gauze mops or squares of old linen or tissues.

NOTE: The temperature of the lotion should be checked in the preparation area.

Bottom shelf

Protective square for bed

Bucket to receive returned fluid

Mackintosh or polythene sheeting to protect floor beneath bucket

Receiver for used rectal catheter or tube

Paper bag for used mops.

NOTE: It is necessary to measure the washout fluid before it is given and also to measure the returned fluid to ascertain that none has been left in the bowel.

9 Enemas

An enema, i.e. an injection of fluid into the rectum, is most commonly ordered either to empty the lower bowel (evacuant enema), or to introduce a medicinal substance for its general or local effect. In the latter case the enema is intended to be retained, if not completely then for as long as possible.

Evacuant Enemas

Disposable

Several proprietary makes of disposable packs of enema solutions, such as sodium phosphate, are available.

A tray with the following equipment is needed:

Disposable enema in container of hot water

Lubricant

Gauze mops, old linen or tissues

Protective covering for bed

Disposal bag

Bed pan and toilet paper should be available

(A suitable sized catheter should be included if the disposable pack nozzle has a jagged edge.)

Soap and Water

A trolley with the following equipment is needed:

Jug containing soap and water solution (280–1120 ml) at body temperature

Funnel
Tubing (approximately 1 m carrying a screw clip)
Connector
Catheter, size 10 or disposable rectal tube
Lotion thermometer
Lubricant
Gauze mops, old linen or tissues
Protective covering for bed
Disposal bag
Bed pan and toilet paper.

While administering an evacuant enema, it is important to observe the patient's condition. If the patient complains of pain or other discomfort, the procedure should be discontinued.

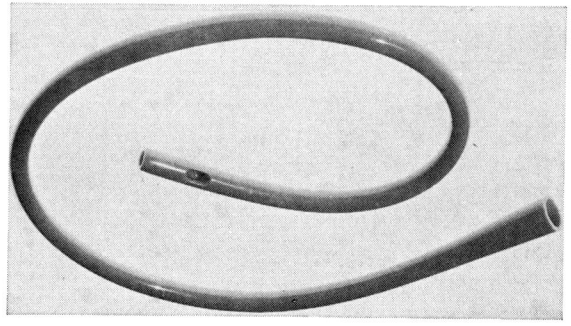

FIG. 36. Rectal tube

Enemas to be Retained

1. A hydrocortisone enema is prescribed for its local anti-inflammatory effect. 100 mg is given in 100 ml normal saline.
2. An olive oil (arachis oil) enema may be prescribed when

it is necessary to soften faeces, e.g. following certain gynaeco-
logical operations. 180–240 ml of warmed olive oil may be
used.

3. A magnesium sulphate enema may be prescribed for the
relief of intracranial pressure. 180–240 ml of a 50% solution
of magnesium sulphate may be used.

These enemas can also be obtained in disposable packs.

4. A resonium enema may be prescribed for a patient who
has hyperkalaemia, and is unable to tolerate oral resonium.
2·6 g of resonium are made into a thin paste with water and
given rectally every four hours.

NOTE: If resonium is constantly administered rectally, it is important that a rectal washout of approximately 1500 ml of
normal saline is given prior to each enema to facilitate the
removal of residual resonium, thus ensuring the maximum
benefit of the pending administration.

To assist the patient to retain an enema, the foot of the bed
should be raised.

Flatus Tube

Passing a flatus tube into the rectum may be ordered for the
relief of abdominal distension due to intestinal gas. This condition may give rise to discomfort post-operatively following
abdominal operations.

A tray with the following equipment is required:

Bowl containing:
    Flatus tube
    Straight glass or plastic connector
    Tubing, approximately 1 m
    Glass or plastic funnel
    Large bowl of water
    Protective square for bed

Lubricant
Container of gauze mops or squares of old linen or tissues
Receiver for used tube
Disposal bag.

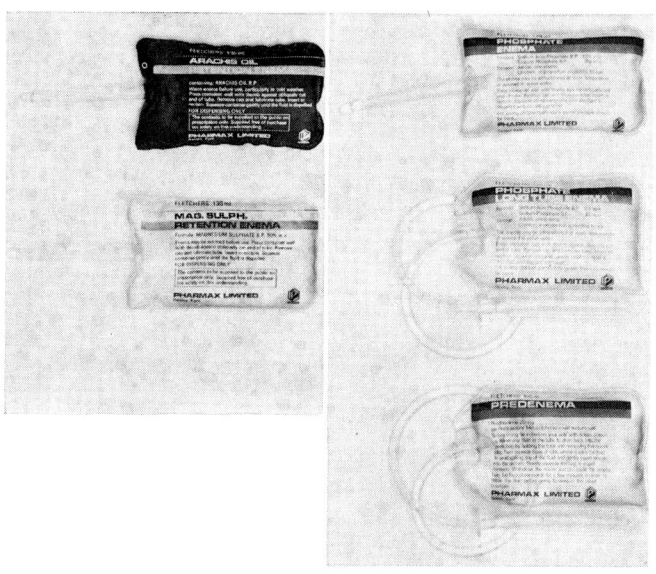

FIG. 37. Examples of evacuant and retainable, disposable enemas

10 Use of Intragastric Tubes

An intragastric tube may be passed for any of the following reasons:

1. To aspirate the stomach contents and empty the stomach in the treatment of acute gastric dilatation or paralytic ileus or prior to an emergency operation.

2. To aspirate the stomach contents for diagnostic purposes.

3. As a method of feeding where the patient is unable to take food by mouth, for example, the unconscious patient, the premature infant who is too feeble to suck, in conditions where there is paralysis of the soft palate or the pharyngeal muscles and following some operations on the mouth, pharynx or larynx.

4. To wash out the stomach in cases of swallowed poisons.

In the majority of cases where an intragastric tube is required, it is passed into the stomach through the nose. When a wide-bore tube is needed, as in gastric lavage for the treatment of poisoning, the orogastric route is used. The nurse must in every case ascertain that the tube is actually in the stomach and this is particularly important before any fluid is poured down an intragastric tube. The omission of this precaution can result in fluid entering the air passages, causing a potentially fatal pneumonia. The usual methods of checking the position of the tube are: (a) Ensuring that sufficient length of tube has been passed to reach the stomach; (b) Opening the mouth of an unconscious patient to make sure that the tube is not coiled up in the oropharynx; (c) Using a syringe to aspirate a sample of the stomach contents.

As a further precaution the aspirated material can be tested with litmus paper. Gastric juice is normally strongly acid and will change the colour of blue litmus paper to red. If there is any doubt about the position of an intragastric tube the nurse should seek help from the ward sister or the medical officer.

Aspiration of Stomach Contents

A tray with the following equipment is needed:

Receiver containing either a suitably sized Ryle's tube or oesophageal tube, adaptor to connect the tube and 20 ml syringe
Litmus paper
Lubricant, e.g. liquid paraffin or glycerine
Container of gauze mops or tissues
Measure jug to receive aspirated fluid
Narrow adhesive strapping and scissors
Cape of protective material or towel
Mouthwash and vomit bowl
Sputum carton and paper tissues
Receiver and paper bag to receive used material.

Some physicians order the tube to be closed with a spigot if it is to be left in position.
Fluid balance chart.

If the tube is passed nasally, a tray holding equipment to clear the nostrils may be required:

Gallipot of wool mops
Gallipot of sodium bicarbonate solution 1 in 160
Receiver containing nasal and dissecting forceps.

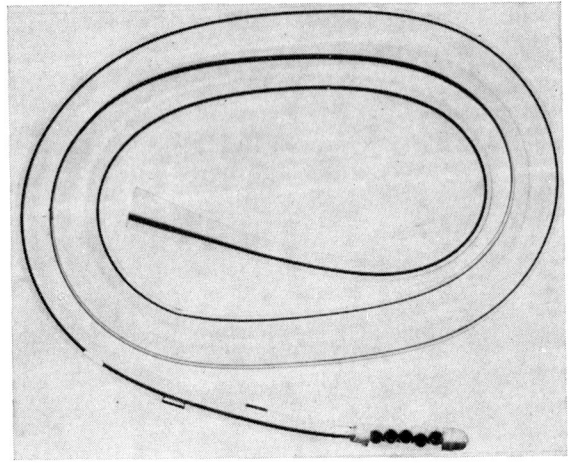

FIG. 38. Ryle's tube

NOTE: The narrow adhesive strapping or a patent tube holder are only required if the tube is to be left in position for further use and should be fixed to the face out of the line of vision.

Pentagastrin Test Meal

The fractional and histamine test meals used for diagnostic analysis of stomach contents have largely been replaced by the pentagastrin test meal. A tray should be set with the equipment to aspirate stomach contents and with the addition of the following:

Pentagastrin (6 μg/kg body weight)
Syringe and needle for subcutaneous injection of pentagastrin

2 specimen containers labelled first and second specimen

Pathology request form

Lotion for cleansing the skin

Mouthwash for use on completion of the test.

Intragastric (Tube) Feeding

The type and quantity of the feed to be prepared will depend on the age and condition of the patient. Usually milk forms the basis of the feeds and the calorie value can be increased by adding sugar or dextrose and cream. An egg and milk mixture or a milk soup may be given and these feeds should be strained. If the tube feeding is continued for more than a few days, 'Complan' or 'Carnation Food'—proprietary preparations containing all essential foods, vitamins and mineral salts —are often used. Alternatively vitamins are added, for example vitamin B complex; and vitamin C, A and D.

If the tube has been left in position, it is necessary to test its position (as previously described), before each feed is given.

Frequent attention must be given to the mouth and careful mouth cleaning is necessary, particularly for the unconscious patient. The conscious patient can use a mouthwash and can also be given chewing gum or pieces of orange to chew and spit out to promote the secretion of saliva, if his condition does not preclude this.

The equipment for aspiration of stomach contents is required, replacing the Ryle's tube by a fine oesophageal tube, and adding the following:

Bowl containing a funnel, short piece of tubing and connector to fit oesophageal tube, gate clip (a syringe with an adaptor may be used to replace funnel)

Measure jug containing feed at body temperature (this jug may be placed in a bowl of warm water to maintain its contents at the required temperature)

A measured quantity of water, e.g. 30 ml

A receiver containing a mouth gag, tongue depressor, wedge and tongue clips are required if the patient is unconscious.

Continuous Intragastric (Tube) Feeding

Equipment is as for aspiration of stomach contents, replacing the Ryle's tube by an oesophageal tube, and with the addition of:

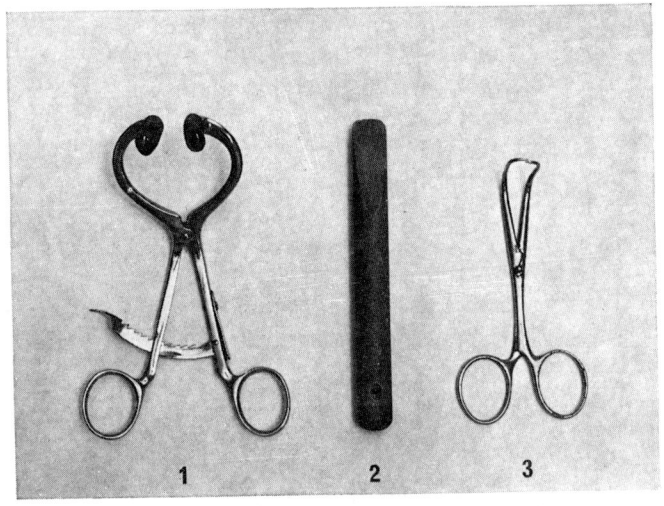

FIG. 39.   1. Mouth gag   2. Wedge   3. Tongue clip

Stand and clip to carry

2 l covered flask or bottle to hold the feed

Bowl containing a short length of tubing to fit bottle or outlet, a drip connection, a longer length of tubing to link this to the oesophageal tube by means of a straight connection

Gate clip

Measure jug containing the feed to be given
Measured quantity of water, e.g. 30 ml
Receiver containing a mouth gag, a tongue depressor, wedge and a tongue clip is required if the patient is unconscious.

Stomach Washout (Gastric Lavage)

Stomach washout may be required in cases of alcoholic poisoning, narcotic poisoning where the poison has been swallowed and aspirin poisoning. It is not usually employed in the treatment of poisoning by caustic or corrosive substances because of the danger of perforating the damaged walls of the oesophagus or stomach. In some cases, however, the Medical Officer may decide to wash out the stomach after neutralizing the poison.

A trolley set with the following equipment is required:

Top shelf
Bowl containing:
    Large oesophageal tube
    Straight connection
    Tubing carrying a screw clip
    Large jug (5 l capacity) of water or prescribed lotion for washout at body temperature
    Small jug to carry washout solution to funnel
    Lubricant, e.g. liquid paraffin
    Container of gauze squares or tissues
    20 ml syringe
    Litmus paper.

Bottom shelf
Cape of protective material or towel
Container for patient's dentures (labelled with patient's name)
    Pail to receive returned fluid

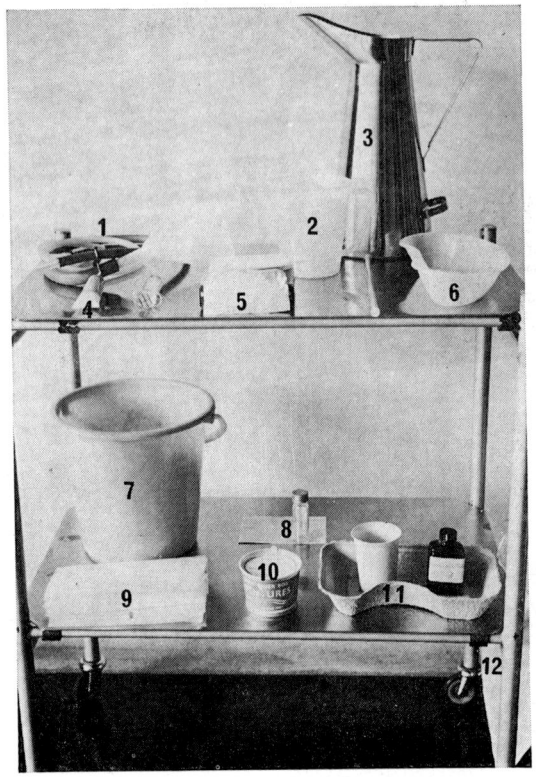

FIG. 40. Equipment for stomach washout

1. Oesophageal tube, connection, tubing and funnel
2. Small jug
3. Large jug for washout solution
4. Lubricant
5. Tissues
6. Receiver containing 20 ml syringe and litmus paper
7. Bucket for returned fluid
8. Specimen jar and pathological request form
9. Protective covering for patient and floor
10. Denture container
11. Mouthwash
12. Paper bag for waste materials

Mackintosh or polythene sheeting to protect floor beneath pail

Paper bag for waste material

Mouthwash for use on completion of washout.

If specimens of the first fluid recovered from the stomach are to be examined, e.g. where poisoning is suspected, two specimen containers, labels and pathological examination forms are required.

A receiver containing a mouth gag, tongue depressor or wooden spatula, wedge and tongue clip are required if the patient is unconscious.

Position of the Patient

A prone or semiprone position with a 'head down' tilt may be used during the washout, especially if the patient is unconscious.

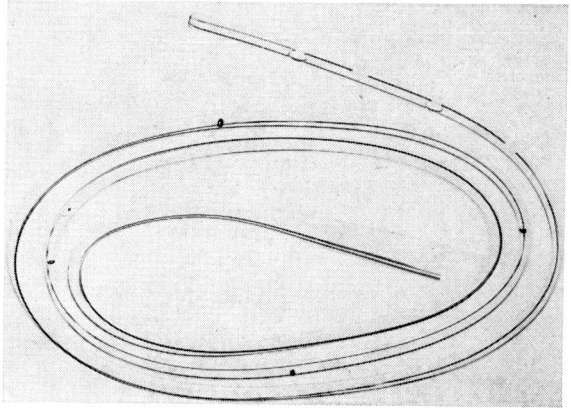

FIG. 41. Stomach tube

11 Examination and Treatment of the Ear, Nose and Throat

Examination

The following equipment is usually provided when the examination is performed in the out-patients' department. The equipment is clean but not usually sterile although it is sterilized after use. For examinations of the nose, throat, or ear in the ward the appropriate instruments would be taken on a tray to the patient's bedside.

Top shelf
  Head mirror
  Containers holding:
    Wooden spatulae
    Wool applicators
    Wool and gauze mops
  Auriscope and aural speculae
  Angled aural forceps
  Wool carrier, e.g. Jobson Horne's probe and wool carrier
or wooden, disposable variety
  Tuning forks
  Nasal speculae
  Local anaesthetic for nasal mucosa, e.g. cocaine 10% solution, cocaine paste 25% strength, cocaine sticks
  Angled nasal forceps
  Straight sinus forceps
  Throat spray of local anaesthetic
  Spirit lamp and matches
  Laryngeal mirrors
  Post-nasal mirrors.

The patient should be provided with 'briefs' to wear and a small blanket should be available to use as needed for warmth during the examination.

The patient's dressing gown and slippers should be nearby, as the physician may wish to see the patient stand or walk.

14 Application of Traction (Extension) to a Limb and Application of Plaster Splints

Traction is most commonly applied to a limb by means of a weight and pulley. In some cases the pull may be obtained by fixed traction with the use of a Thomas's splint.

Traction may be used as an interim measure in the treatment of fractures of the lower limb, but is more usually employed in the treatment of fractures of the femur and to prevent deformity and relieve pain in diseases of the joints, such as arthritis and tuberculous infection.

The treatment may also be applied by skeletal traction, when a pin or a wire is inserted through the bone and the weight is hung on to this by means of a cord attached to a metal horseshoe (spreader) or by skin traction when adhesive strapping is applied to the skin and the weight is attached to a spreader which may be incorporated in the strapping or connected to it, by webbing and buckles or by cord being passed through the strapping. Methods vary from one hospital to another. The insertion of the pin or wire is a procedure carried out in the operating theatre with full aseptic precautions and using the preparation required for all bone operations.

Skin Traction

The following equipment is required:

Top shelf
    Requirements for shaving the limb
    Tape measure
    Zinc oxide plaster extension kit (child or adult)
    Sorbo rubber or Zopla felt
    Scissors.
    Tincture Benzoin (Friar's Balsam) may be required to paint
the skin before the application of the extension plaster. If this
is to be done a small paint brush or forceps and wool mops
will be needed to apply the Tinc. Benz. Co. or a proprietary spray (Rikospray).

Bottom shelf
    Thomas's splint
    Calico bandages (10 cm or 15 cm)
    Bulldog clips
    Safety pins
    Extension cord
    Weights or graduated water bags, plus a carrier
    2 Crepe bandages
    Bed blocks to raise foot of bed if ordered
    Extension fitting for end of patient's bed
    Small blanket and sock
    Gamgee padding to cushion the leg.

Ventfoam Skin Traction Bandage

This form of traction may be ordered when a weight of not
more than 4·5 kg is required, or occasionally when traction
is a very temporary form of treatment. It is used for very

young children and adults who cannot tolerate zinc oxide plasters and where there is possible danger of the breakdown of skin. Ventfoam should be checked daily and re-applied as and when necessary.

A tray containing the following equipment is required:

Ventfoam bandage (proprietary pack) 5, 7·5 or 10 cm width
Spreader provided with proprietary pack
4 crepe bandages
Safety pins or zinc oxide tape
Extension cord
Extension fitting for end of patient's bed
Bed blocks to raise foot of bed
Weights or graduated water bags and carrier.

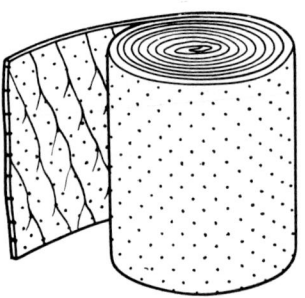

FIG. 48. Ventfoam bandage

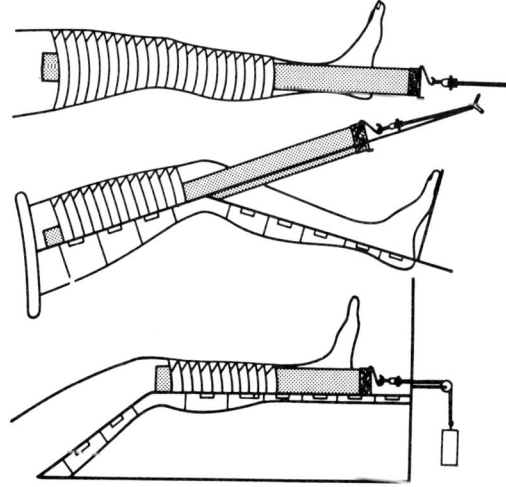

FIG. 49. Ventfoam bandage in use

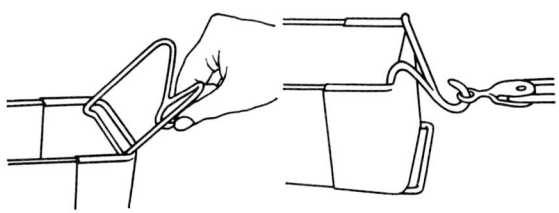

FIG. 50. Spreader bar

Plaster of Paris Splints

Splints made of muslin bandages impregnated with plaster of
Paris (anhydrous calcium sulphate), are very widely used in
the treatment of fractures and in orthopaedic surgery. They
have advantages over most other types of splints in that they

are inexpensive, accurately fit the part to which they are applied and once applied do not need constant readjustment.

'Gypsona' plaster proprietary bandages are commonly used but occasionally bandages may be prepared by the nursing

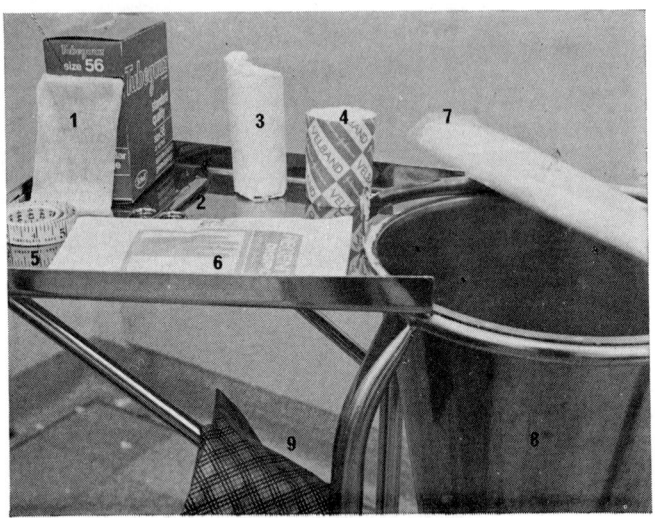

FIG. 51. An arrangement of the equipment for the application of Plaster of Paris

1. Roll of stockinette
2. Plaster scissors
3. Plaster bandage
4. Cotton wool bandage
5. Tape measure
6. Rubber gloves
7. Mackintosh
8. Bowl of tepid water
9. Plastic apron

staff. The material used is either book muslin or butter muslin, cut into strips 3 or 4 m long. The most useful widths are 7·5, 10, 15 and 20 cm. Loose threads are removed and the muslin strips loosely rolled or folded. The dry plaster is then rubbed into the meshes of the muslin as evenly as possible, using the palm of the hand rather than the fingers. As each successive length of the bandage is impregnated with the plaster it is loosely rolled up. A coloured thread may be run across the width of the free end of the completed bandage, thus making the end easier to find when the bandage is removed from the bowl of water ready for use.

Plaster bandages should be stored in airtight tins. They are immersed in tepid water sufficiently long to soak the entire thickness of the rolled bandage and until all bubbles have subsided. Only one bandage is soaked at a time.

Application of Plaster of Paris

A trolley is required containing the following equipment:

Roll of stockinette (diameter of part to be treated)
Sorbo or Zopla felt (if moulding is required)
Cotton wool or foam bandages
Plaster bandages correct size for part being treated
Plaster scissors and tape measure
Deep bowl of tepid water
Plastic apron and rubber gloves for operator
Mackintosh to protect patient and floor.

15   Inhalations

Inhalations may be dry or moist and are used in the administration of drugs and treatment of respiratory diseases.

The administration of oxygen may be of benefit to patients whose respiratory capacity is diminished for any reason. Oxygen may, for example, be ordered following chest injuries or operations, in pneumonia, cardiac failure, and acute pulmonary oedema.

Dry Inhalations

OXYGEN should always be used with extreme care, as it can become a danger to the patient if used indiscriminately.

Precautions to be Observed when Oxygen is in Use

1. Prohibit the use of the following in the immediate vicinity: (a) matches, cigarette lighters, cigarettes, pipes, cigars and naked flames from any source; (b) electrical appliances, e.g. electric shavers, electric bells, portable radios; (c) sparking or mechanical toys should not be allowed.

2. Place a 'NO SMOKING' notice on the cylinder.

3. Warn visitors of precautions against fire.

4. Do not grease fittings and joints on cylinders and flow-meters.

5. Store cylinders in cool place.

6. Check further supplies when cylinder in use is one quarter full.

The basic equipment for the administration of oxygen is as follows:

Source of oxygen:
Wall point from a pipe line, or oxygen cylinder (black base, white top) in stand, fitted with a flowmeter and pressure gauge and a spanner to open the cylinder
'NO SMOKING' notice
Antistatic pressure tubing to connect the source to the apparatus used to administer oxygen.

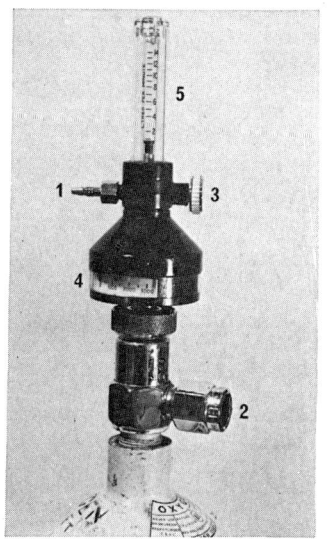 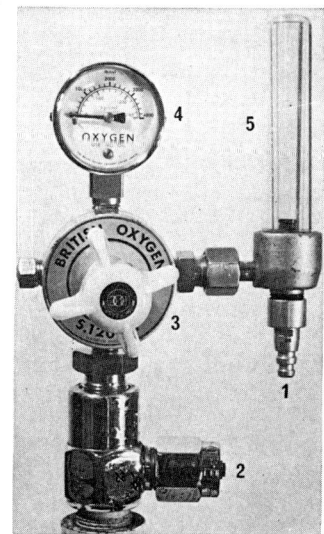

FIG. 52. Oxygen cylinders

1. Outlet (tube to mask or spectacles is attached here)
2. Main control valve
3. Fine adjustment valve

4. Gauge showing amount of oxygen in cylinder
5. Flowmeter showing rate at which oxygen is leaving cylinder

Administration may be by proprietary disposable mask, e.g. 'Venti' mask (*Oxygenaire*).

Administration may be by disposable nasal spectacles or nasal catheters.

A special type of disposable mask is available for a patient who is to receive oxygen via a tracheostomy tube.

If the nostrils are crusted, equipment to cleanse them before beginning oxygen therapy will be required as follows:

Small tray containing:
  Gallipot of wool swabs
  Gallipot of sodium bicarbonate solution 1 in 160
Receiver containing 1 pair nasal and 1 pair dissecting forceps
Paper bag for used mops.

A humidifier is also required. This is attached to the source of oxygen by a short piece of pressure tubing and oxygen is carried from the humidifier by the pressure tubing connected to the mask or spectacles. The humidifier must receive constant, thorough cleansing, as it may become a source of pathological micro-organisms which are then inhaled by the patient.

Administration by Means of an Oxygen Tent

The manufacturers of these tents are constantly modifying and improving their equipment. In each case the maker's instructions should be studied in order to provide the necessary equipment. In addition to the basic equipment, a supply of ice may be required. Where the tent does not cover the whole bed, a drawsheet is used to secure the front edge of the canopy. The end of the canopy can be rolled in this and the ends of the drawsheet tucked under the mattress to prevent any leak of oxygen from the tent.

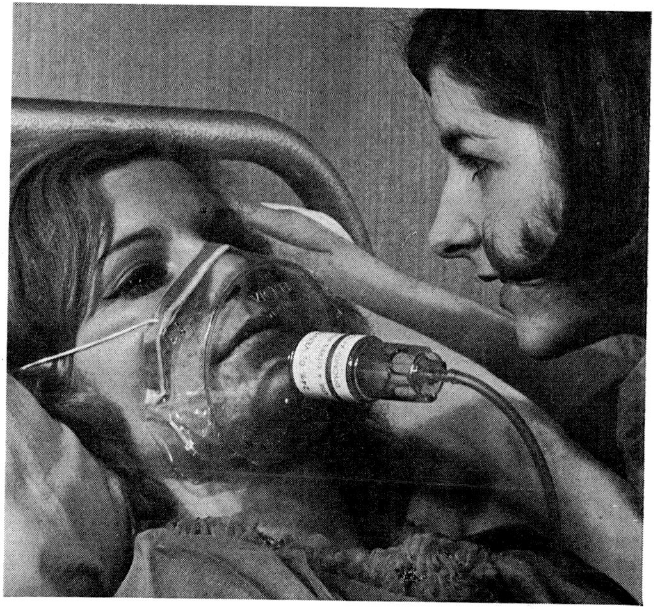

FIG. 53. 'Venti' mask in use

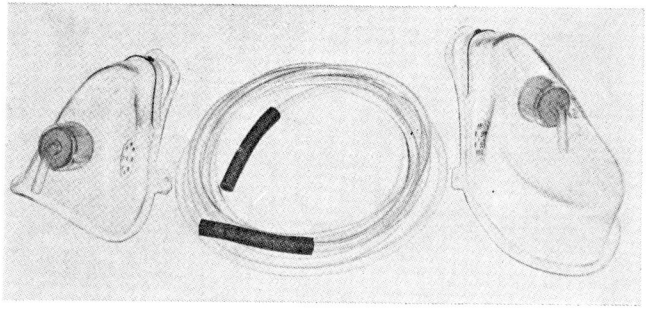

FIG. 54. Oxygen tubing and disposable face masks

Care of the Patient

Patients having oxygen therapy should be under the continual observation of the nursing staff. The apparatus must be frequently and carefully checked; should the oxygen supply fail the patient may be unable to get sufficient air from other sources. Patients who develop pneumonia superimposed on chronic bronchitis and emphysema may become mentally confused, with muscular twitching and a full bounding pulse during oxygen therapy. This condition is known as carbon dioxide narcosis. Such patients are usually ordered intermittent rather than continuous oxygen therapy.

DRY INHALATIONS in the form of *capsules or sprays*, produce a vapour which is inhaled by the patient, e.g. to relieve spasm of bronchial tubes in asthma or for the relief of chest pain as in angina pectoris.

The capsules are broken in gauze or a clean handkerchief and the vapour inhaled.

The spray is dispensed through a nebulizer and sprayed directly into the patient's mouth for inhalation.

Moist Inhalations

In the treatment of upper respiratory congestion, e.g. sinusitis or catarrh, the open jug method is preferable. For lower respiratory infection, e.g. bronchitis, the Nelson's inhaler is used.

A tray containing the following equipment is required:

Nelson's inhaler or 1 l jug
Prescribed amount of Tinc. Benz. Co. (Friar's balsam) or menthol

Boiling water
Bowl to stand inhaler in
Gauze to protect mouthpiece
Tissues
Sputum mug
Cover for inhaler
Disposal bag
Spoon.

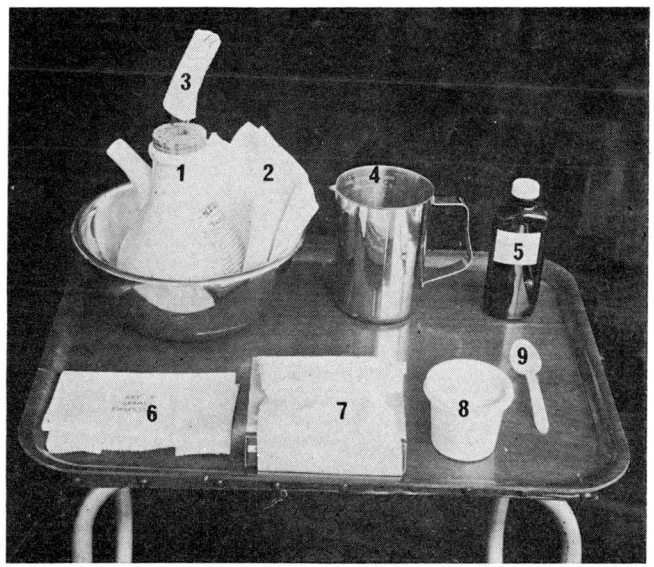

FIG. 55. Moist inhalation

1. Nelson's inhaler
2. Cover for inhaler
3. Gauze for mouthpiece
4. Jug for boiling water
5. Tinc. Benz. Co.
6. Disposal bag
7. Tissues
8. Sputum mug
9. Spoon to measure medication

Care should be taken to ensure the patient is fully coopera-
tive. The patient is kept in an even temperature throughout
treatment.

Some patients may derive benefit from being nursed in a
warm moist atmosphere, e.g. when a tracheostomy has been
performed, and in the absence of the modern sophisticated
humidifier, a steam kettle may be used in conjunction with a
canopy which has been erected over the patient's bed. If the
patient is being nursed in a single-bedded room the canopy
is unnecessary.

16   Sponging

Sponging may be ordered for the reduction of temperature by up to 1 °C in the febrile patient or for a sedative effect in the case of a patient who is uncomfortable and restless even if his temperature is only moderately raised.

Where tepid sponging is ordered the temperature of the water used should be between 21 °C and 26 °C (70–78 °F). Sponging with iced water may be necessary in hyperpyrexia where the patient's temperature is 40·5 °C (105 °F) or over. Where the treatment is given mainly for its soothing effect and the patient complains of aching muscles and a tender skin, a hot sponge with water at a temperature of 40·5 °C (105 °F) may be more comforting than a tepid sponge.

The following equipment will be required:

Top shelf
Washing bowl of water for sponging at the required temperature

Washing bowl of cold water to cool sponges being used in turn

Marine sponges, 2 large and 4 small if available, or pieces of soft towelling

Small bowl of iced water

Material, e.g. lint, for compress for patient's forehead

1 jug of cold water to correct the temperature of the water as necessary.

Clinical thermometer if this is not available at patient's bedside

Bath thermometer.

Bottom shelf
    2 bath blankets
    Hairbrush and comb
    Clean nightwear
    Clean bed linen
    Temperature and pulse record chart
    Drink of iced water or fruit juice
    Face cloth and face towel
    Where the procedure is ordered to reduce body temperature,

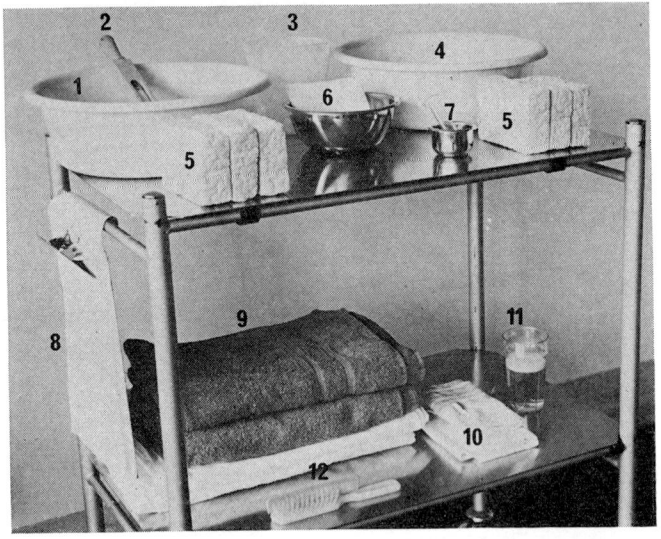

FIG. 56. An example of a trolley set for tepid sponging

1. Bowl of tepid water
2. Thermometer
3. Jug for cold water
4. Bowl of cold water
5. Sponges
6. Bowl of iced water and compress
7. Clinical thermometer
8. Record chart
9. Bath blankets and clean bed linen and nightwear
10. Face towel and flannel
11. Iced drink
12. Hairbrush and comb

the patient's pressure areas are treated by changing the position rather than the application of lotions and powder since the associated friction is undesirable. Where the procedure is ordered for its soothing effect, then requisites to treat the pressure areas may be added.

Care of the Patient

Throughout the procedure for tepid sponging, the patient should be observed carefully for indications of a rapid fall in temperature which may be a complaint of feeling cold, shivering or signs of developing rigor. If such signs present themselves, the treatment should be stopped, the patient covered and the temperature taken.

17 Local Applications

Cold Application

Proprietary packs of chemicals ('dry ice') may be used for the application of cold. These are simply prepared by placing in a refrigerator as directed on the pack. They may be used repeatedly and it is then usual to label the pack with the patient's name and to place it in a small tray when refreezing. The tray may be used to carry the pack to the patient and can then be sterilized.

A local cold application such as an ice bag or a 'dry ice' pack may be ordered to prevent swelling, for example in the treatment of such injuries as sprains or bruising, to arrest haemorrhage and may be used for the relief of headache.

The following equipment is required to apply an ice bag:

Poultice board or a convenient working surface may be used
Ice pick or large safety pin
Ice
Piece of old flannel to contain ice being broken
Bowl to contain ice chips
Metal spoon in jug of hot water (this is used to stir the chips —the heat removes any sharp edges)
Ice bag or a polythene bag of the required size, Sellotape to seal the open end and a cover
Cloth to dry ice bag
Salt and teaspoon (some hospitals make a practice of adding a teaspoonful of salt to the ice in the bag and consider

it increases the cooling power of the ice by its action of lowering its melting point)

Where the ice bag is to be suspended, a cradle and cotton bandage are required

A tray to carry the ice bag to the patient.

NOTE: The area of application should be observed at frequent intervals to ensure frostbite does not occur (shown by mottling of the skin).

Application of Heat

Kaolin Poultice

A clay or kaolin poultice is applied for the relief of pain in inflammatory conditions. It may be used in the treatment of pneumonia and pleurisy. It may also be ordered in the early stages of such local inflammations as a boil or carbuncle.

The basis of the application is china clay, to this are added glycerin and a counter-irritant such as methyl salicylate.

The following equipment is required:

Poultice board or a convenient working surface

Old linen or white lint large enough to cover affected area

Palette knife to apply kaolin to linen or lint (a spatula is used if palette knife is not available)

Container of kaolin standing in the saucepan of water in which it has been heated

Single layer of gauze which may be used to cover the poultice

2 warm plates or bowls to carry poultice to bedside

Piece of cottonwool a little larger than the poultice, bandage and pins to secure poultice in position

Paper bag to receive previously applied poultice if necessary.

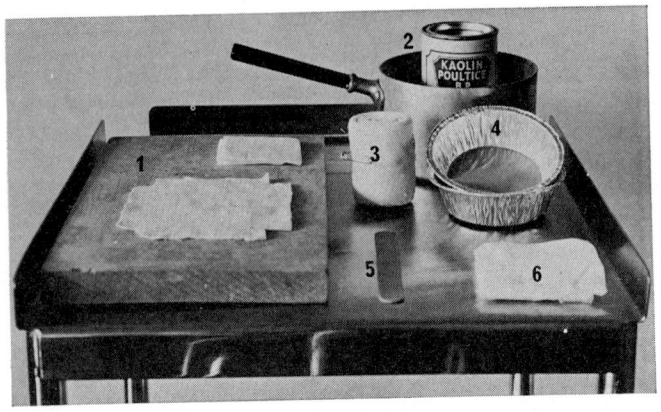

FIG. 57. A tray showing equipment for the application of a kaolin poultice

1. Poultice board with white lint and gauze
2. Saucepan containing tin of kaolin
3. Bandage
4. Plates or bowls to carry poultice
5. Wooden spatula
6. Cotton wool

18   Last Offices

When death has taken place and the relatives have left the bedside, all top bedclothes should be removed with the exception of the sheet, which is left to cover the body. Check that the identity bracelet is in position, written legibly, and leave on. The body should be placed straight in the bed with the feet together and the hands at the side. Close the eyes; if necessary cover with a moist wool swab or place a wisp of wool under the eyelids to keep them closed. Place cleaned dentures in position. The mouth is closed and jaw supported by a bandage or a small pad placed under the chin. Any jewellery should be removed unless the relatives have expressed a wish that it should remain on the body. The pillows, air-ring and any treatment trays that have been used should be removed from the bed and locker. The nurse then prepares a trolley for the laying-out. Where possible two nurses should carry out this office for an adult patient. A second washing bowl and the necessary articles for washing the body may be set on another trolley or tray, or one nurse may wash as the second nurse dries the body.

The following equipment is required:

Top shelf
   Washing bowl of warm water
   Washing cloth and soap
   Nailbrush and nail scissors
   Two bath towels
   Hairbrush and comb
   Shaving requisites for men

A tray containing:
    Sinus forceps
    Dissecting forceps
    White wool
    Non-absorbent wool
If the deceased has a dressing in place add 2 pairs dressing forceps, gauze squares and waterproof strapping.

NOTE: Stitches are NOT removed but it is usual to remove any drainage tubes and to close the opening with gauze securing this with wide waterproof strapping.

Bottom shelf
    Shroud
    Mortuary sheet
    Identification labels
    Notification of Death forms
    Receiver containing safety pins, clips or needle and cotton if these are customarily used to secure mortuary sheet
    Paper bag to receive used disposable material
    Container to receive used forceps
    Containers to receive any catheters or transfusion equipment removed
    Valuables and property, books
    Bag and label (for personal effects).

NOTE:
    1. Advice should be sought regarding patients that have received treatment by a radioactive source prior to death. In some hospitals a 'radioactive' label is attached to the body before leaving the ward area.
    2. The coroner's officer may need to be notified in the event of a patient dying through certain circumstances, e.g. road traffic accident, or sudden death by an unknown cause.

In these cases, advice should be sought before performing last offices.

3. Certain religious sects prefer to make their own arrangements regarding last offices for deceased relatives and such wishes should be respected.

Glossary of Instruments

This glossary is designed to show the detailed appearance of some of the instruments illustrated in the text which on account of their small size may not be seen sufficiently clearly in the photographs. A few pieces of apparatus in addition to those depicted in the trays and trolleys have also been included where it was considered that this might be helpful.

A short description of each instrument and its uses has been given, as this may help the nurse to memorize the different patterns, especially if the distinguishing features of each are noted and their purpose realized. For instance, the illustrations of the various types of forceps show clearly the differences in their blades and the manner in which they grip, and this will aid the nurse in learning their names and the purposes for which they are required.

Adaptors

Adaptor

A short connection, usually made of metal, used to unite two pieces of apparatus of different bore, e.g. to connect a piece of rubber tubing to a needle or cannula, or to connect a needle to the nozzle of a syringe.

(1) **Adaptor** to fit syringe.

(2) **Two-way adaptor** and stop cock.

(3) **One-way adaptor** and stop cock.

Auriscope

Auriscope

An instrument designed for facilitating the inspection of the auditory meatus and the drum of the ear. The term auriscope is usually used to distinguish between the ordinary aural speculum and the electric auriscope which is illuminated by a small bulb, the power being supplied by a battery in the handle of the instrument.

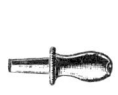

Adaptor

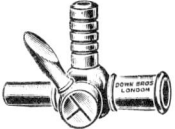

Two-way
adaptor

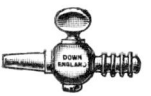

One-way
adaptor

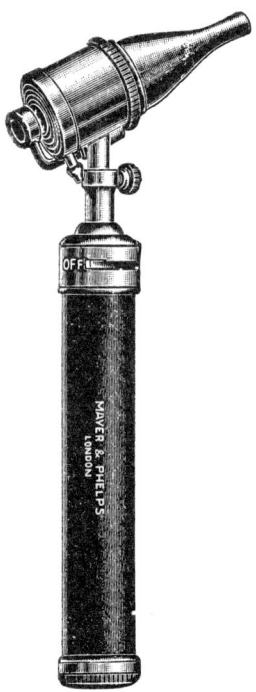

Auriscope

Catheters

Catheter

A hollow instrument which may be made of metal, rubber or plastic, designed for withdrawing urine from the bladder. The term is also used for similar instruments introduced into other cavities or passages of the body, e.g. **Eustachian catheters**, which are passed into the Eustachian tube connecting the nasopharynx and the middle ear, and **ureteric catheters**, used for exploring the ureters and draining the pelves of the kidneys.

Indwelling Catheter

One which is intended to remain in the bladder for some period; an ordinary urethral catheter may be tied in or a **self-retaining** type of catheter may be used, e.g. a Jaques catheter

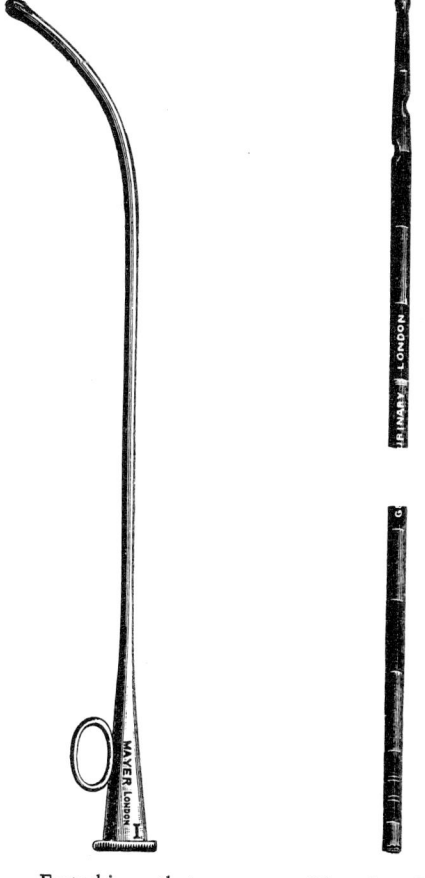

Eustachian catheter   Ureteric catheter

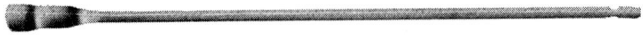

Jaques catheter

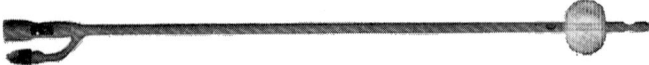

Jaques catheter showing inflated balloon

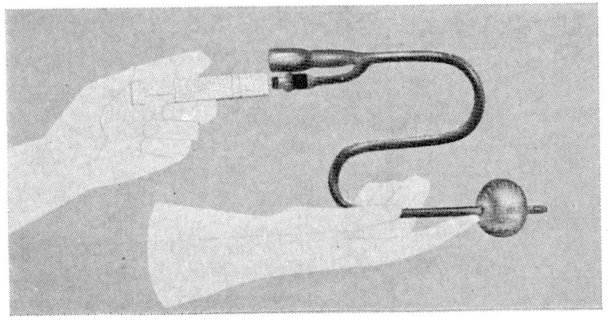

Operator inflating balloon

Clips

Tubing Clips

Tubing clips are obtainable in different sizes and patterns according to their use. The simple spring type of clip (1) is used for clipping the tubing of such apparatus as is used for giving irrigations or enemas after the tubing has been filled with fluid to expel air.

The Mayo Clinic pattern clip (2) is easily and quickly manipulated.

The screw pattern (3) is useful when it is necessary to use the clip to regulate the rate of flow of fluid through a piece of tubing as, for example, in connection with the apparatus used for giving 'drip infusions'.

Wound Clips

Metal clips are used for closing the skin in place of, or in addition to sutures. The usual type of metal clip used is the Michel clip (4). Special forceps are required to compress the clips bringing together the skin edges of the wound.

Towel Clips

Small cross-action or clip forceps are used to clip sterile towels and so retain them in position.

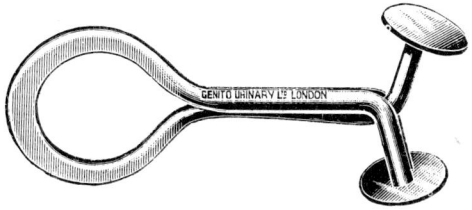

(1) Tubing clip (Mohr's)

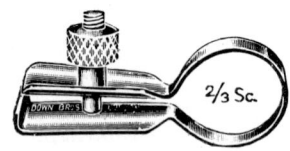

(2) Tubing clip (Mayo clinic pattern)

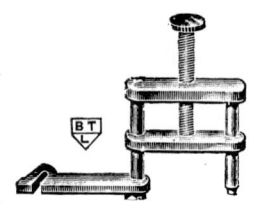

(3) Tubing clip (screw pattern)

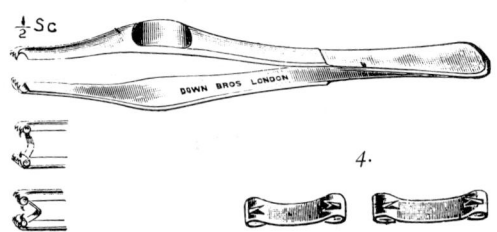

(4) Michel's clips and clip-compressing forceps

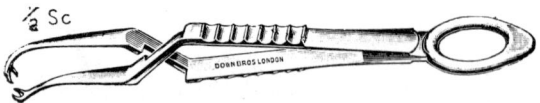

Towel clip (cross-action)

Dilators

Dilator

An instrument used for dilating an opening.

(1) **Rectal dilator.**
(2) **Vaginal dilators.**
(3) **Tracheal dilator.**

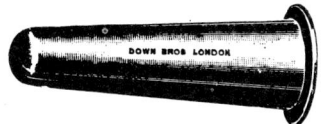

Perspex rectal dilator

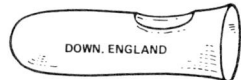

Glass vaginal dilator

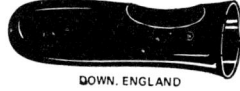

Vulcanite vaginal dilator

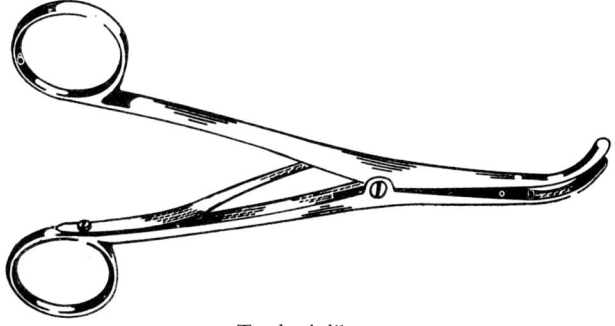

Tracheal dilator

Forceps

Forceps

Instruments used for holding dressings and other surgical apparatus and for grasping or compressing tissues. (Some of the forceps mentioned are shown on p. 116.)

(1) **Artery forceps.** Spencer Wells's pattern, Kelly's 'mosquito' fine artery forceps.

(2) **Clip-removing forceps**, Michel's.

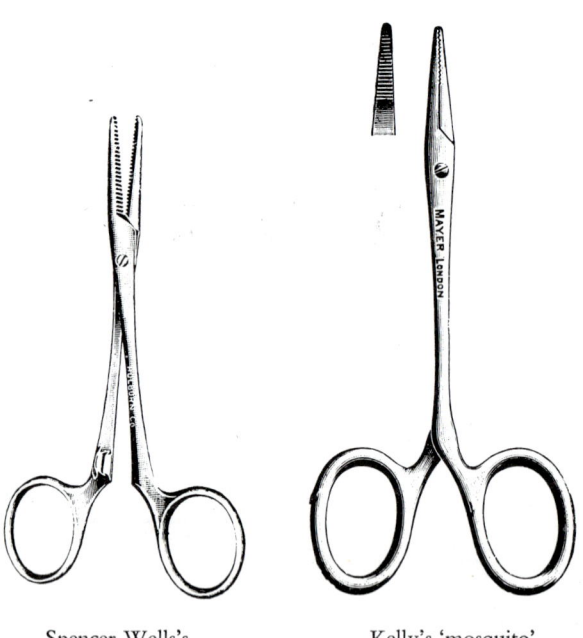

Spencer Wells's
artery forceps

Kelly's 'mosquito'
artery forceps

(3) **Dissecting forceps**. Used for dissecting tissues and for handling dressings; plain and toothed blades.

(4) **A needle-holder**. The type shown, which is in very common use, is a pair of catch forceps with grooved blades.

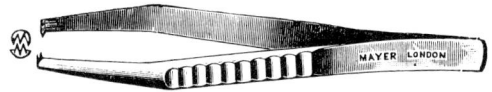

Toothed dissecting forceps

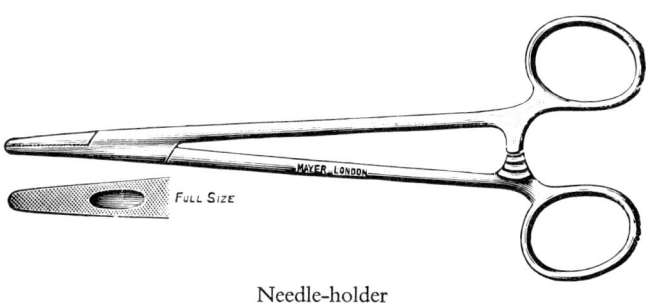

Needle-holder

(5) **Dressing forceps**. Used for holding swabs, (A) angular dressing forceps, (B) nasal dressing forceps, (C) French pattern dressing forceps, (D) long-handled sponge-holding forceps used for swabbing cavities such as the throat and the vagina.

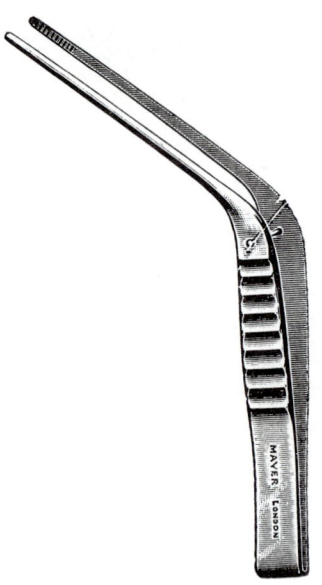

(A) Angular dressing
forceps

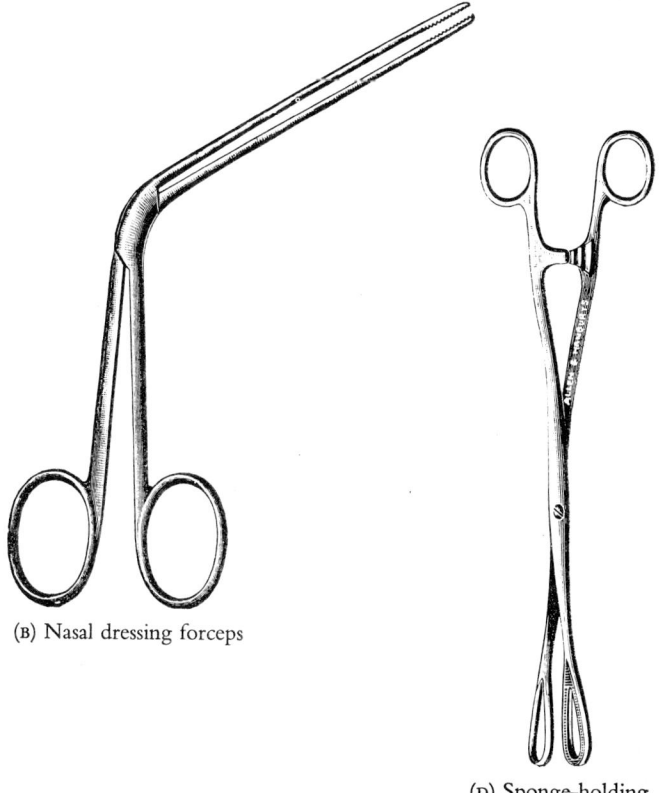

(B) Nasal dressing forceps

(D) Sponge-holding forceps

(6) **Sinus forceps.** Used for opening up a sinus or for introducing a drainage tube or gauze plugging into a sinus or a cavity.

(7) **Tongue forceps.** For grasping the tongue and pulling it forward.

(8) **Sterilizer forceps** (Cheatle's). Long-handled forceps used for removing instruments and apparatus from boiling water and for handling sterile equipment.

(9) **Tissue-grasping forceps.** Lane's tissue forceps, catch forceps with fenestrated blades. Volsellum forceps with claw blades, commonly used for holding the cervix of the uterus.

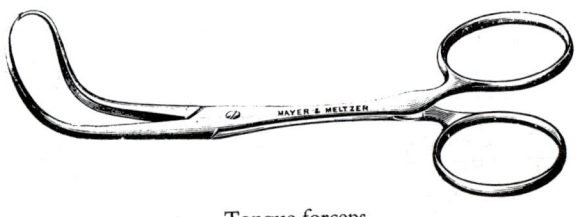

Tongue forceps

Lane's tissue forceps

Cheatle's
sterilizer
instrument
forceps

Volsellum forceps

Gags

Gag

An instrument used for opening the mouth and keeping it open in order to help maintain an airway during the administration of an anaesthetic, or during the clonic stage of a fit when the patient may bite his tongue. A gag may also be required to open the mouth of an unconscious patient in order to clean the mouth, or to pass a tube for a stomach washout or for a tube feeding.

The two types illustrated are the gags most often used in the ward.

(1) **Ferguson's gag.**

(2) **Doyen's gag.**

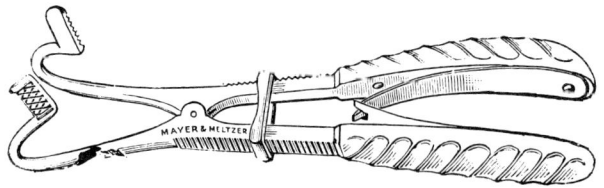

Ferguson's gag

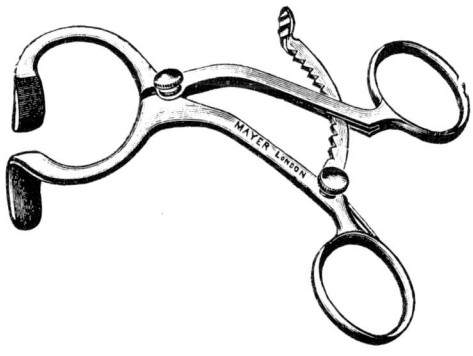

Doyen's gag

Mirrors

Mirror

Used in conjunction with a light, which is reflected in the mirror.

(1) **Head mirror** is strapped to the operator's forehead, and is used to reflect light into aural or nasal orifices.

(2) **Laryngeal mirror** used in examination of the throat.

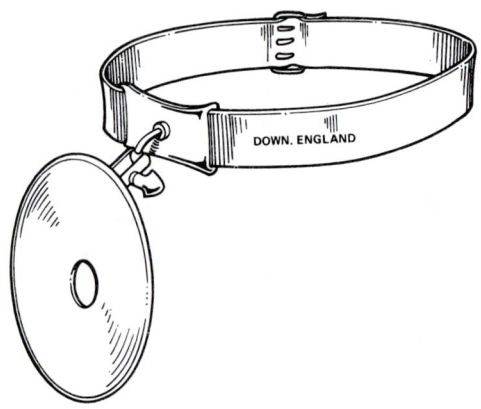

Head mirror

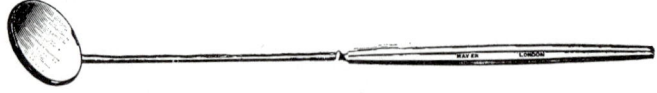

Laryngeal mirror

Needles

Needles

Needles are made in various sizes and shapes according to the purpose for which they are designed.

(1) **Suture needles**

    (a) Straight triangular.

    (b) Curved triangular.

    (c) Triangular half-circle.

The needles illustrated are those most often required for procedures carried out in the ward, as, for example, suturing the incision made in cutting down on a vein.

(2) **Aneurysm needle**. A blunt needle on a handle used for passing a ligature under a vessel, as, for example, under the vein in the operation of cutting down on the vein for transfusion purposes.

(3) **Hollow needles** used for injections and also for the withdrawal of fluid from the body.

    (a) **Hypodermic needle**, size 17, the needle most commonly used for hypodermic injections.

    (b) **Gordh's intravenous injection needle**. This needle can be left *in situ* and is useful when repeated injections have to be given.

    (c) **Sternal puncture needle.**

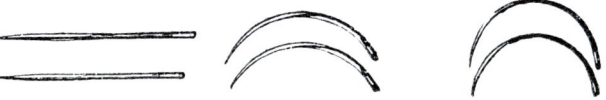

(A) Straight triangular (B) Curved triangular (C) Triangular half-circle

Suture needles

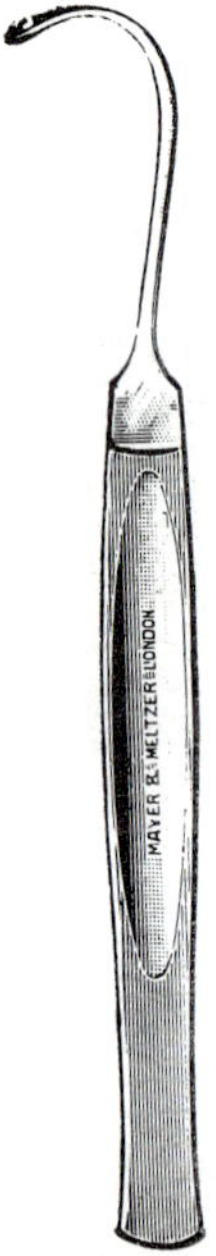

Aneurysm
needle

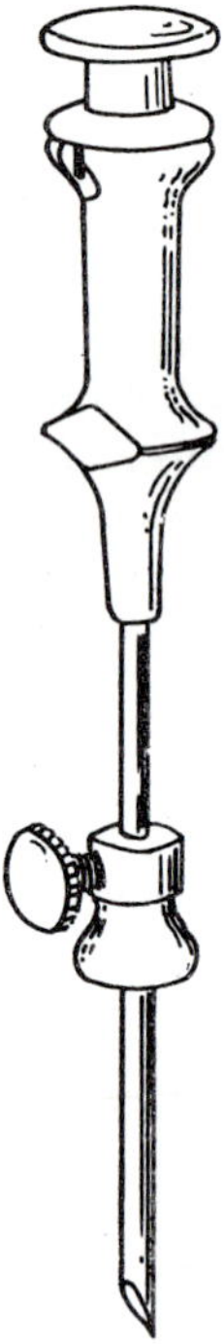

(c) Sternal
puncture needle

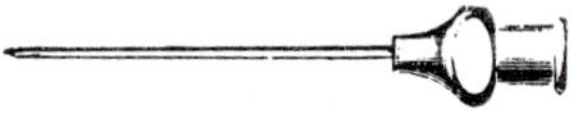

(A) Hypodermic needle
size 17

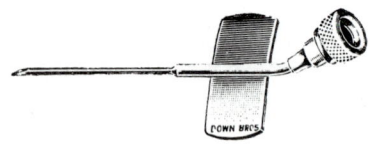

(B) Gordh's intravenous injection needle

Pessaries

Pessary

An instrument used for supporting a displaced uterus. The pessary is introduced by insertion into the vagina.

(1) **Ring pessary.**
(2) **Ring pessary introducer.**
(3) **Hodge pessary.**

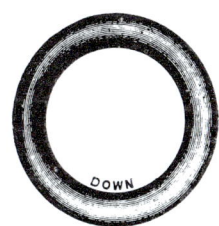

Ring pessary

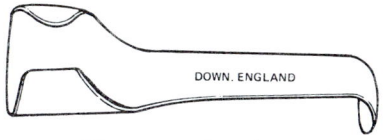

Ring pessary introducer

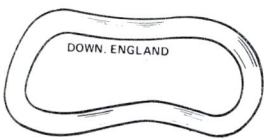

Hodge pessary

Probes

Probe

An instrument used for exploring a cavity, wound or sinus; also used as an applicator when dressed with cotton wool.

(1) **Wound probe** (see p. 16).

(2) **Probe, director and raspatory.**

(3) **Jobson Horne's probe.** Probe with ring end and wool carrier used for removing wax from the auditory meatus.

(4) **Intrauterine probe and applicator.**

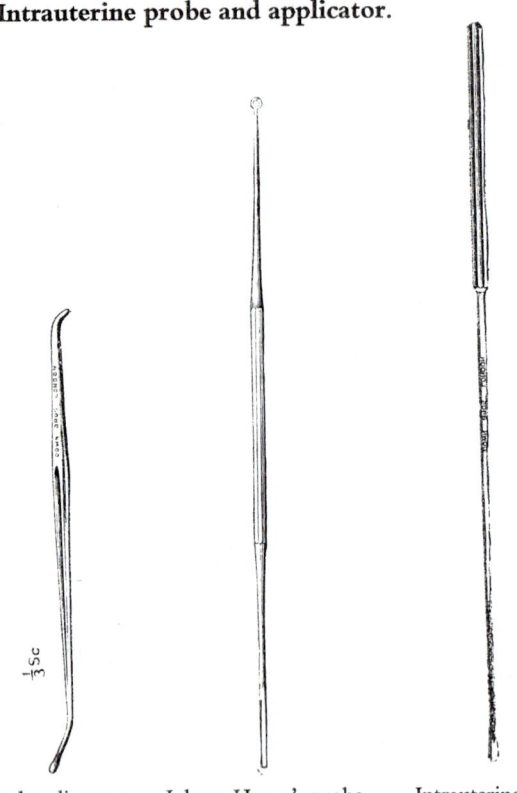

Probe, director   Jobson Horne's probe   Intrauterine probe
and raspatory   and wool carrier   and applicator

Scraper

Scraper

This instrument is a wooden one, used to collect specimens of
cervical tissue for pathological examination.

(1) **Ayre surface biopsy scraper.**

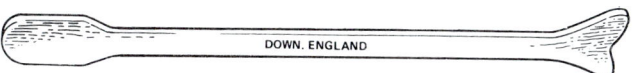

Ayre surface biopsy scraper

Sounds

Sound

A solid cylindrical instrument, curved or straight, for exploring a hollow cavity
   (1) **Bladder sound.** (A) male, (B) female.
   (2) **Uterine sound.**

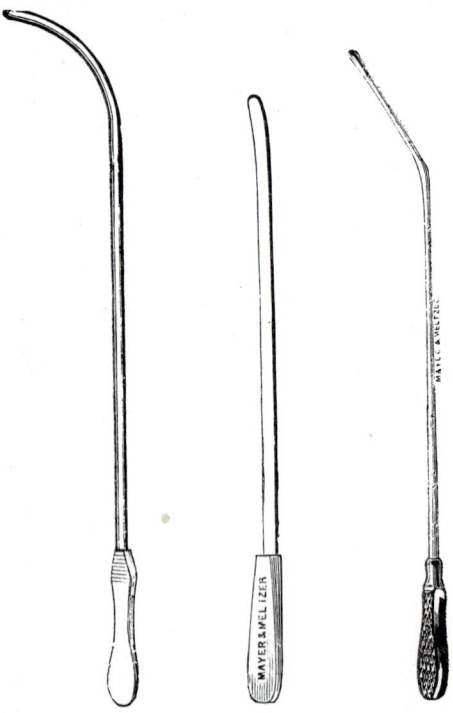

(A) Male bladder   (B) Female   Uterine
   sound   sound   sound

Syringes

Syringes

Syringes of various patterns are used for irrigations and injections.

(1) **Aural syringe**.

(2) **Higginson's syringe**. For attachment to the cannula for irrigating the maxillary antrum.

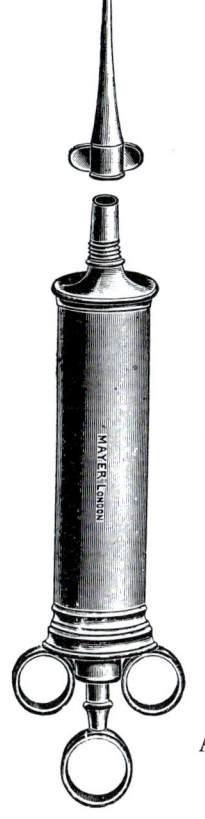

Aural syringe
capacity
120 ml.

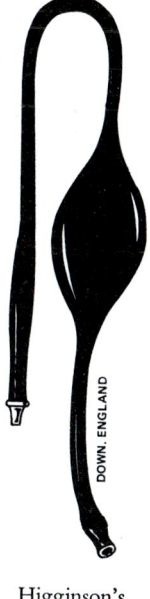

Higginson's
syringe

Specula

Speculum

An instrument for enlarging the opening of a cavity or keeping a passage patent, thus facilitating inspection.

(1) **Aural speculum**.
(2) **Nasal speculum**.
(3) **Rectal speculum** or proctoscope.
(4) **Vaginal speculum**.

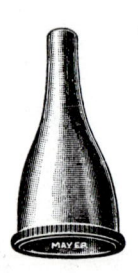

Aural speculum

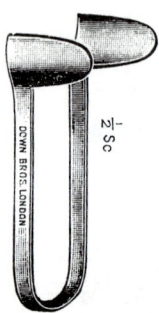

Nasal speculum

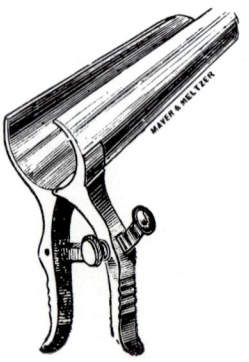

Rectal speculum

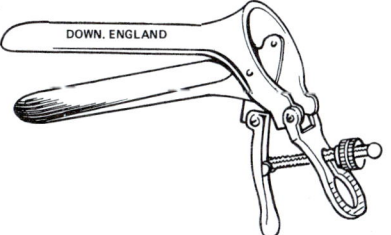

Cusco's vaginal speculum

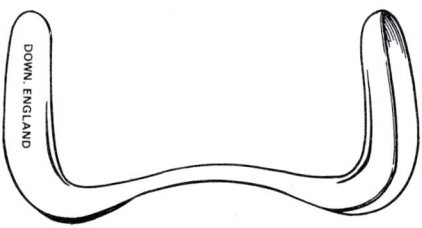

Sims' duckbill speculum

Illuminating Specula

Perspex specula are obtainable fitted with an electric light to illuminate the cavity to be inspected.

The photographs show:

(1) A 'Coldlite' illuminated **bivalve vaginal speculum.**

(2) A 'Coldlite' illuminated **proctoscope**, or rectal speculum.

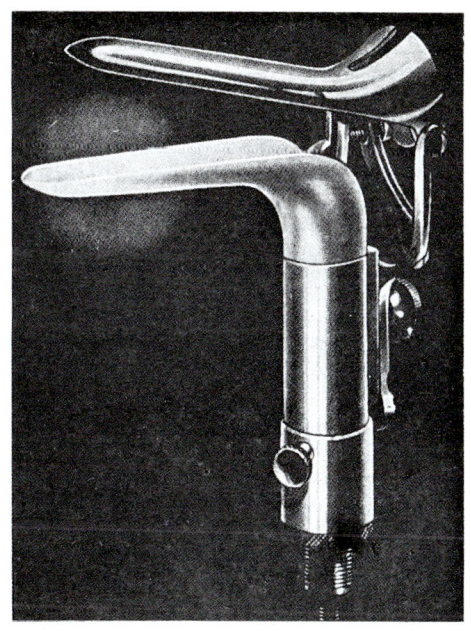

Bivalve vaginal speculum

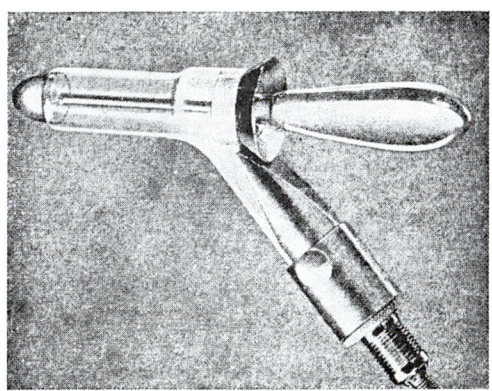

Proctoscope

Tongue Depressors

Tongue Depressor

Tongue depressor, used to control the tongue during examination of the throat, or during the routine care of a patient's mouth.
  (1) **Straight glass** tongue depressor.
  (2) **Straight stainless steel** tongue depressor
  (3) **Angled** tongue depressor.

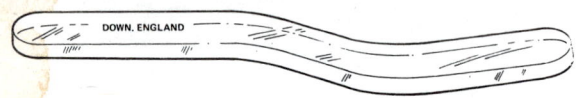

Straight glass tongue depressor

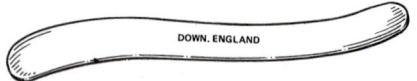

Straight stainless steel tongue depressor

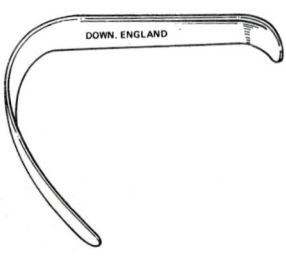

Angled tongue depressor

Tracheostomy Tubes, Laryngostomy Tube, and Tracheal Dilators

Tracheostomy tubes are metal, rubber or plastic tubes inserted through an incision in the neck into the trachea in order to maintain an airway when the larynx is blocked by a foreign body, by swelling, by pressure or by diphtheritic membrane. A tracheostomy may also be required prior to operations on the larynx or pharynx or in cases of laryngeal or pharyngeal paralysis or before treatment of this area by radiotherapy.

The artificial opening may be required for a short period only, or it may (especially in malignant disease) be a permanent one.

(1) **Parker's tracheostomy tube**. This tube is made in nine sizes, and for children may be preferred to the Durham's tube.

(2) **Baker's india-rubber tracheostomy tube.** This tube may be used for a permanent tracheostomy once a sinus is established.

(3) **Butlin's laryngostomy tube** and introducer.

As an emergency operation in adults, laryngostomy may be undertaken as an alternative to tracheostomy.

(4) **Bowlby's tracheal dilators**. A pair of dilators should be kept on the trolley at the bedside of every tracheostomy case, not only for use when the outer tube is changed, but also as a means of keeping the trachea open if the outer tube should accidentally slip out of the trachea.

(5) **Disposable tracheostomy tube.** This tube is made of plastic or P.V.C. and is used when the tracheostomy is a temporary one. It is discarded after use.

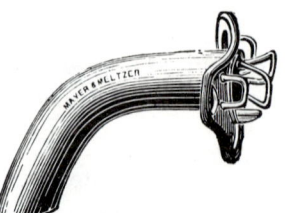

Parker's tracheostomy tube

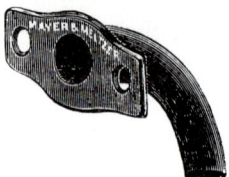

Baker's india-rubber tracheostomy tube

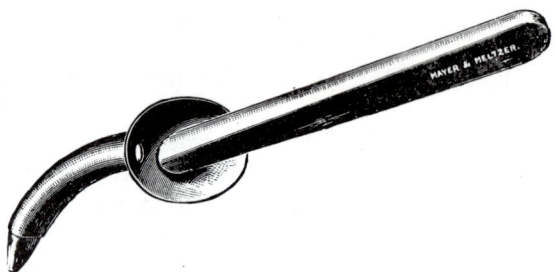

Butlin's laryngostomy tube

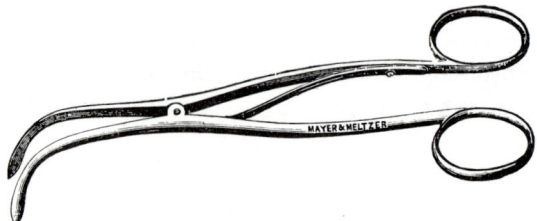

Bowlby's tracheal dilators

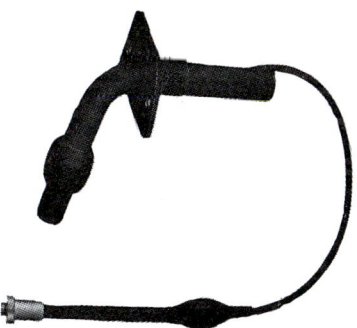

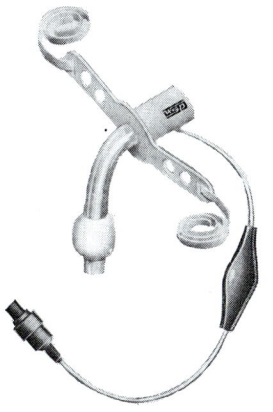

Disposable tracheostomy tubes

Tuning Fork

Tuning Fork

A metal instrument used for testing hearing by means of the sounds produced by its vibration.

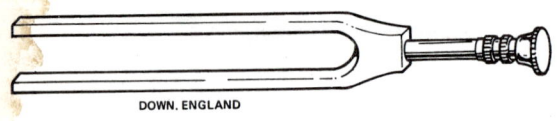

DOWN. ENGLAND

Tuning fork

Index